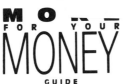

A MORE
FOR YOUR
MONEY
GUIDE

Freebies (& More) For Folks Over Fifty

$

Linda Bowman

PROBUS PUBLISHING COMPANY
Chicago, Illinois

Library of Congress Cataloging in Publication Data Available.

ISBN   1-55738-218-2

Printed in the United States of America

BB

1   2   3   4   5   6   7   8   9   0

TABLE OF CONTENTS

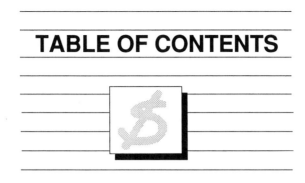

CHAPTER 2
SPORTS, FITNESS, AND EXERCISE FOR SENIORS

INTRODUCTION

HAVE THE TIME OF YOUR LIFE
IN THE PRIME OF YOUR LIFE

This book is for those of you who know you are on the threshold of what should and can be the very best years of your lives. There are over 62 million Americans over the age of 50. You are as varied, active, interesting, vital and exciting as any group can be. However, as a group, there are only two things you have in common:

1. You were born before 1940.

2. You have earned admittance into the incredible, wonderful, wide world of "freebies" and special discounts for folks over 50.

Because of the variety in your interests, abilities, and activities, and the differences between the segments within the 50+ age group, there is no name or label that properly identifies everyone. The new definition of "middle age" has been set between the years of 44 and 66. Since that is the case, forget the idea of "senior." Most of you are still enjoying the "prime of your life": middle age. For the sake of simplifying terms, we will use "mature adult" and "senior citizen" interchangeably through-out this book, hopefully satisfying the majority of our readers, whether they have just turned 50 or are nearing 90. Since most mature adults claim to feel on the average, 15 years younger than their chronological age, labels have become nearly meaningless.

Along with the problems of labeling folks 50 and over are the false assumptions and stereotypes that sometimes accompany those labels:

1

- Mature adults are all the same.
- Mature adults are always becoming ill and suffer from poor health.
- Mature adults are set in their ways, stubborn, and difficult.
- Mature adults have nothing to contribute to society.
- Mature adults are draining our country of its funds.
- Mature adults are weak and non-influential, as individuals and as a group.
- Mature adults should be retired at age 65.
- Mature adults are poorer than other segments of the population.
- Mature adults are basically lonely.
- Mature adults lose their mental faculties and can't think or reason as well as they used to.
- Mature adults prefer the company of older people like themselves.
- Mature adults are physically inactive and become more sedentary as they get older.

We could go on, but be aware that all of the above statements and any others you've heard are entirely false, foolish and without substance. In fact, in every case the reverse is true:

- You can actually be healthier, happier, and live longer now than ever before.
- Your financial situation can be significantly better and continue to improve after you reach 50.
- Your relationships and friendships can be deeper and more meaningful than before. Romance can even get better with experience, time, and maturity on your side.
- Your health can remain excellent and you can participate in nearly any physical activity you choose.

- Your mental faculties can be sharper, your senses keener, and your beliefs and needs more focused than they were in your youth.

- Your choices are greater than ever, with more time on your hands and the freedom to do what you want whenever you want.

- You can achieve goals you've always aspired to, rising to new levels of knowledge and ability. Learning and becoming are processes that live as long as you do.

- You can make an important difference in the quality of your life and the lives of all mature adults.

- You alone, have the ability and wisdom to cross generational barriers and communicate, teach, and reach out to others of all ages.

Mature adults are the fastest growing segment of the population, representing nearly a quarter of the people in the United States today. As a result the business community is intensely aware of the purchasing power held by mature adults. With over $900 million in combined annual income and $160 million in discretionary income, seniors as consumers are a formidable force. In addition, the dozens of senior organizations, associations and advocacy groups representing millions over the age of 50, are no longer ignored by our leaders and lawmakers on Capitol Hill. Meeting the growing needs and demands of this group will continue to be a significant challenge in the future.

The products and service areas that focus on the mature market with discounts and privileges continue to grow yearly as the number of seniors continues to increase. Some of the areas offering freebies, discounts and great deals that we discuss in this book include:

- *Transportation:* airlines, car rentals, trains, buses.

- *Entertainment:* concerts, movies, theater, attractions, theme parks, restaurants, sports events, fairs, museums, zoos, aquariums, historical sites.

- *Sports:* Senior Olympic and multi-sport competitions, tennis, golf, swimming, walking, skiing, cross-country skiing, dancing, running, biking, bowling.

- *Shopping:* chain department stores, bookstores, toy stores, home repair services, automobile repair services, medical and dental services, gasoline service stations.

- *Travel:* cruises, tours, travel clubs, hotels, motels, resorts, free travel, adventure travel, package deals, national parks and recreation areas, travel with grandchildren.

- *Financial investments, savings and insurance:* bank and S&L discounts and perks, retirement and investment advice, free insurance information, tax advice.

- *Education:* travel/study programs, free and low-cost adult education programs, college and university programs, computer networking for seniors.

- *Health:* health screenings, free information, treatment, preventative programs, medicine and prescription drugs.

These topics include some of the major concerns and interests of mature adults. In addition we've included some helpful suggestions and guidelines to aid you in getting these deals and enjoying them as much as possible.

There are some terrific opportunities out there waiting for mature adults. Savings can be found nearly everywhere you look. Not only can you save when you're having fun (which is where most people think all the savings are), but you can save at your bank, where you shop, going back to school, and in your health care needs. You can save from $1 to thousands of dollars, from 10 percent to 90 percent by being aware and informed of the hundreds of special senior privileges, discounts, and perks available just because you've turned 50. Some of the freebies and good deals that we've included are available to all age groups—not just seniors. We just want to make sure you're aware of them.

To take advantage of these deals, all you need to do is ask for them. The two most important questions to ask, now that you're part of the mature market, are:

1. **"Do you have discounts for seniors?"**

2. **"What is the lowest available rate?"**

Memorize these questions and use them everywhere you go to purchase products and services. Soon you will be realizing savings you never thought possible. And they weren't, before this. You have entered a new life and a new world. They say life is a series of "passages." Today being 50 and older means passing through the wide doors of enjoying the best things in life. So why not enjoy them for less and even for free?

WELCOME TO THE WORLD OF SENIOR SAVINGS AND HAVE THE TIME OF YOUR LIFE IN THE PRIME OF YOUR LIFE!!

CHAPTER 1

LET US ENTERTAIN YOU (FOR LESS!)

One of the most exciting and diverse areas for great senior deals and discounts is the area of entertainment. Wherever you go to have a good time and enjoy yourself, you can probably do it for less than the price listed, and sometimes even for free. Some of these attractions and entertainment opportunities include:

> movies, dances, concerts, theme parks, museums, historic sites, theaters, restaurants, tourist attractions, sports events.

Always ask about a senior citizen discount before buying a ticket or paying an entrance fee. It's not always advertised that such discounts are available. You should always carry your driver's license (or other proof of age I.D.) or membership card in an over-50 club as proof that you deserve a break. A lot of folks who have kept fit and healthy through the years simply don't look 50 or 55 and may be asked for proof of age.

MOVIES AND CONCERTS

Free movies and concerts are some of the most enjoyable events offered nearly everywhere, often on a weekly or monthly basis at the same location. Senior centers, libraries, museums, and public auditoriums make use of their empty spaces and community rooms during the day by running classic movies, educational movies, or special movie series.

There are also free daytime concerts given by musical groups who volunteer their talents in the community. (For example, summer concert series and holiday musical performances in shopping centers and malls.) Parks and recreation departments also sponsor free events (often aimed at retirees and those who are free from daily jobs and family obligations) such as dances and concerts given by local school bands, dance, and music departments.

Many of the performers themselves are retired professionals or working professionals who still perform regularly at "paying" events. These concerts give those who can't afford the steep price of tickets a chance to experience quality musical events.

For example, the following free events were recently listed in our local senior newspaper:

FREE MOVIES—Classic films Saturdays, Aug. 11 & 18, 6 & 8 P.M.; Sundays, Aug. 12 & 19, 11 A.M. & 1 P.M., West Hollywood Park Auditorium, 647 N. San Vicente.

FREE MOVIES—Frank Capra's award-winning films, Fridays, 7-10 P.M., through Aug. 3. Ebell Theater, 1100 E. Third St., Long Beach.

SUNDAYS AT FOUR—Free chamber music series, each Sunday, 4 P.M., Bing Theater, L.A. County Museum of Art, 5905 Wilshire Blvd.

FREE CONCERTS—Tuesdays, 6-7 P.M., beginning June 19 with Verdugo Swing Society, Memorial Park Bandshell, Raymond and Walnut St., Pasadena. June 26—Dixieland.

In addition to classics, if you like first-run movies, you can nearly always save money off the adult ticket price. Senior citizen discounts for movies range from 25 to 75 percent off regular ticket prices. With tickets approaching $7 per adult, this is an important discount if you enjoy going out to the movies.

FAIRS AND EXPOS

Festivals, expos, state and county fairs, circuses, and special-interest shows also offer discounts for seniors. In addition, auto shows, house and garden shows, antique shows, holiday fairs, ski shows, recreational vehicle shows, travel shows, arts and crafts shows, gift shows, and even air shows often have senior discounts on admission prices.

EAT FOR CHEAP (OR FREE)

Over the past several years, the restaurant industry has found it pays to be good to their older patrons who are among the largest percentage of repeat customers. As we know, from fast food chains to four-star establishments prices have been rising steadily. Since 1978, eating out has increased by 6 percent overall, but it has increased more than 20 percent among adults 50 and over.

A simple way to eat for cheap, in fact for free, is to patronize restaurants that have special "Happy Hours." These are held during the slow times (usually betwen 4 and 6 P.M.), when restaurants are looking for business before the normal dinner hour. As incentive, these restaurants offer specially priced drinks and free hors d'oeurves. We have seen some tables filled with hot and cold free hors d'oeurves that would easily make a tasty meal, and a filling one at that. "Happy Hours" are very popular at Mexican restaurants where the selection of goodies is quite large.

Restaurants with popular bars often feature a delicious array of free food that often changes nightly. Although you have to order a drink, it needn't be an alcoholic one. Juices and soft drinks will do quite well. And the delicious rewards on the hors d'oerves table are well worth the price. (By the way, if you are a football fan, don't forget "Monday Night Football." Look for bars and restaurants with large-screen televisions that advertise "free" food for coming in to watch the game and have a drink.)

"Early Bird Dinners" and "Sunset Meals" are especially popular with budget-minded diners who value quality food at good prices. Generally, a main course, vegetable, dessert, and beverage are included at a price lower than what the main course alone would cost during regular hours. Although they apply to everyone, they are targeted to seniors who often prefer to eat their evening meal early (sometimes making it their main meal of the day). We found that most restaurants offer these specially priced meals until 6:30 or 7:00 P.M.

Many individual restaurants offer senior citizen discounts on regular menu items or have a special senior menu with lower prices. Some feature two for one senior dinners. You can usually find these specials in the restaurant section of your daily newspaper or senior publication. If you're not sure whether a restaurant has a senior special, ask for it.

Several national and regional restaurant chains offer senior citizen discounts (at all hours). A few, like Denny's, are especially interested in the preferences and concerns of their older patrons. And for good reason: Adults over 55 make up nearly one-third of all of Denny's customers patronizing their 1,200 restaurants around the country. Depending on the individual restaurant chain's policy, discounts may be identical everywhere or may differ slightly from location to location. The restaurant may issue "membership" cards valid at all locations to seniors who patronize them frequently. Here are some examples of senior discounts at large chains:

1 POTATO 2 offers a 10 percent discount on any purchase for those over 62. Sixty-five outlets throughout United States and Japan.

ARBY'S offers a 10 to 20 percent food discount, a free beverage with meal, and free coffee. Age requirements may vary from 55 to 60 and over depending on management's program. Not every location offers the discount program.

DENNY'S has a Senior Menu, which includes smaller portions for breakfast, lunch, and dinner items. There is also a nightly dinner special that changes every day.

HOLIDAY INN restaurants give Mature Outlook members 10 percent off their food bill. Those belonging to the Holiday Inn Travel Venture Club also receive food discounts.

RED LION INNS and THUNDERBIRD MOTOR INNS will give card-carrying members of AARP, Mature Outlook, and Silver Saver's Passport a 15 percent discount on regularly priced food items.

BOB'S BIG BOY family restaurants offer 10 percent off any meal, at anytime for anyone in a party that includes one person over 55. Bob's Big Boy Senior's Discount Cards are valid at all participating restaurants.

SIZZLER restaurants Senior Club members (55 and older) are entitled to 20 percent off any regular menu item every day from 2 to 5 P.M., and all day Monday, Tuesday, and Wednesday. They also have a Senior Menu with light and lean items.

INTERNATIONAL HOUSE OF PANCAKES recently offered seniors a "limited time only" coupon offer of a complete special dinner for just $3.99 after 4 P.M.

MR. STEAK has a "Senior Diner" program that gives a 10 percent discount (before taxes) on regularly priced meals at restaurants displaying a "Senior Diner" symbol.

TASTEE FREEZ INTERNATIONAL has determined that older folk are the number one consumers of dipped ice cream and gives a 10 percent discount to its "Gold Club" members at participating locations around the country.

TCBY frozen yogurt stores offer seniors the "Golden Discount Program" giving them 10 percent off the price of a single menu item and 20 percent off items through promotional mailing programs.

DUTCH PANTRY restaurants (located in PA, DL, NC, OH and WV) give senior citizen discounts of 10 percent off all regular menu prices.

RAX restaurants give senior citizen discounts of 10 percent on all items on their menu. Rax has approximately 400 outlets around the country.

SAVINGS AT UNUSUAL RESTAURANTS

Some combination dinner/theater attractions also give seniors a break including:

ARABIAN NIGHTS DINNER ATTRACTION in Kissimmee, Florida. 10 percent senior citizen discount off $25.94 regular adult admission. AARP members and guest receive $20.94 senior citizen admission. Tel: (800) 553-6116.

HORNBLOWER DINING YACHTS. Operate in California harbors. 10 percent senior citizen discounts on all regularly scheduled dining cruises. Tel: (800) 950-0150

MEDIEVAL TIMES, Kissimmee, Florida, and Buena Park, California. Jousting knights dinner attraction. 10 percent senior citizen discount off $26 + tax regular adult price. Tel: (800) 327-4024.

M.S. DIXIE, Lake Tahoe, California dinner cruises. $15.50 senior citizen cost (regular cost, $19.50).

WESTGATE DINNER THEATER, Toledo, Ohio. $18.75-$25.75 senior citizen rates ($19.75-$26.75 regular adult prices) Tel: (419) 536-6161.

TOURIST ATTRACTIONS

Most tourist attractions around the country give special rates to senior visitors. Members of local or regional senior citizen organizations and clubs may also be entitled to special savings off entrance fees. Many attractions advertise special "limited time only" discounts for seniors at certain times of the year. These special promotions are often lower than the regular senior discounts. Some well known U.S. attractions that offer senior citizen discounts include:

BOOT HILL MUSEUM, Dodge City, Kansas. (316) 227-8188.

COLONIAL WILLIAMSBURG, Williamsburg, Virginia. (804) 229-1000.

CORAL REEF STATE PARK, Key Largo, Florida. (800) 432-2871.

THE EMPIRE STATE BUILDING, New York, New York. (212) 736-3100.

GATORLAND, Orlando, Florida. (407) 855-5496.

GRAND CANYON CAVERNS, between Kingman and Seligman, Arizona. (602) 422-3223.

METEOR CRATER, Flagstaff, Arizona. (602) 774-8350.

NBC STUDIOS TOUR, Burbank, California. (818) 840-3549.

NEW ORLEANS STEAMBOAT COMPANY, New Orleans, Louisiana. (800) 365-BOAT.

PALM SPRINGS AERIAL TRAMWAY, Palm Springs, California. (619) 325-1391.

QUEEN MARY AND SPRUCE GOOSE, Long Beach, California. (213) 499-1629.

SANTA'S WORKSHOP, North Pole, New York. (518) 946-2211.

THE UNITED NATIONS, New York, New York. (212) 963-7713.

UNIVERSAL STUDIOS, Orlando, Florida. (407) 363-8000, Hollywood, California. (818) 777-3762.

All three major television networks invite viewers to see their favorite shows for free taped at their studios. To receive tickets, send a self-addressed stamped envelope to: NBC Tickets, 3000 W. Alameda Blvd., Burbank, CA 91523; CBS Tickets, 7800 Beverly Blvd., Los Angeles, CA 90036; ABC Tickets, 4151 Prospect Ave., Hollywood, CA 90027

VISIT A MAGIC KINGDOM FOR LESS

People of all ages are fascinated by amusement and theme parks. For most of us, one visit is never enough. We love going with our children, our grandchildren, our friends, and of course, out-of-town guests. Most amusement parks offer senior citizen discounts. Of particular note is the Disney Magic Years Club, which entitles those over 60 to year-round reduced prices at both Disneyland and Walt Disney World. They also are good for discounts on parking, meals, shops, some Hilton Hotels, and National Car Rental locations. Members also receive a quarterly newsletter and vacation packages at Walt Disney World, Disneyland and other locations. A lifetime membership costs just $25.

A sampling of other major amusement/theme parks that offer senior discounts include:

ADVENTURE ISLAND, Tampa, Florida. (Ask about the Club 55+ Discount Card) (813) 988-5171.

ATLANTIS THE WATER KINGDOM, Hollywood, Florida. (305) 926-1001.

BUSCH GARDENS, Tampa, FLorida. (Ask about the Club 55+ Discount Card) (813) 988-5171.

CEDAR POINT, Sandusky, Ohio. (419) 626-0830.

THE GREAT ESCAPE FUN PARK, Lake George, New York. (518) 792-6568.

HERSHEYPARK, Hershey, Pennsylvania. (800)-HERSHEY.

KINGS ISLAND, Kings Island, Ohio. (513) 398-5600.

KNOTT'S BERRY FARM, Buena Park, California. (714) 827-1776.

LIBERTYLAND AMUSEMENT PARK, Memphis, Tennessee. (901) 274-1776.

MARINELAND OF FLORIDA, Marineland, Florida. (904) 471-1111.

MARINE WORLD AFRICA USA, Vallejo, California. (707) 644-4000.

RAGING WATERS, San Dimas, California. (714) 592-8181.

RIVERFRONT PARK, Spokane, Washington. (509) 456-5512.

RIVERSIDE AMUSEMENT PARK, Agawam, Maine. (800)922-7488.

SEA LIFE PARK HAWAII, Waimanalo, Hawaii. (808) 259-7933.

SEA WORLD, San Diego, California, (619) 222-6363; SEA WORLD of Ohio, Aurora, Ohio, (800) 63-SHAMU. SEA WORLD of Texas, San Antonio, Texas. (512) 523-3000.

SIX FLAGS OVER MID-AMERICA, Eureka, Missouri, (314) 938-5300; SIX FLAGS MAGIC MOUNTAIN, Valencia, California, (818) 367-2271; SIX FLAGS OVER GEORGIA, Atlanta, Georgia, (404) 948-9290.

WATERWORLD USA, Phoenix, Arizona. (602) 266-5200, WATERWORLD USA BIG SURF, Tempe, Arizona. (602) 947-SURF.

WATCH AND WAGER FOR LESS

The races (dog and horse) are another exciting pastime that is popular among mature adults. Race courses around the country offer senior discounts, free "senior days," "senior matinees," and "half-price" senior discounts. A few tracks offering discounts include the following (check your local race courses for discounts):

CHURCHILL DOWNS, Louisville, Kentucky. (502) 636-4400.

DAYTONA BEACH KENNEL CLUB, Daytona Beach, Florida. (904) 252-6484.

EARL WARREN SHOWGROUNDS, Santa Barbara, California. (805) 687-7598.

MEADOWLANDS RACETRACK, East Rutherford, New Jersey. (201) 460-4054.

NORTHEAST FLORIDA KENNEL CLUBS, Jacksonville, Florida. (904) 646-0001.

SANTA ANITA PARK, Arcadia, California. (818) 574-RACE.

IF YOU'RE LOOKING FOR CULTURE

From art, science and industry, natural history, and sports museums to zoos, botanical gardens, planetariums, and historical landmarks, seniors will find a wide array of educational and cultural attractions that offer senior discounts throughout the year. They are found in every city in the country, rural areas, and out-of-the-way places. Astounding, awesome, and breathtaking, the treasures, beauty, and experiences of these places will fill your days with wonderful and lasting memories.

Besides the fact that many government-run institutions and estab-lishments admit seniors for free (including rides, special exhibits, trans-portation and events inside the attraction), these places offer interesting and stimulating insights into how this country was founded and built. Check with individual organizations for pertinent information including days and hours, senior discounts, "free" days, wheelchair access, current exhibits and special programs, membership information and services, guided tours, etc. Remember, always ask for your discount and present your identification before paying admission.

ABBY ALDRICH ROCKEFELLER FOLK ART MUSEUM, Williamsburg, Virginia, (804) 229-1000.

ARLINGTON NATIONAL CEMETERY, Arlington, Virginia, (703) 683-2007.

BERKELEY MUNICIPAL ROSE GARDENS, Berkeley, California, (415) 644-6530.

BETSY ROSS HOUSE, Philadelphia, Pennsylvania, (215) 627-5343.

BIRMINGHAM MUSEUM OF ART, Birmingham, Alabama, (205) 354-2565.

CALIFORNIA AFRO-AMERICAN MUSEUM, Los Angeles, California, (213) 744-7432

CALIFORNIA MUSEUM OF SCIENCE AND INDUSTRY, Los Angeles, California, (213) 744-7400.

CALIFORNIA STATE CAPITOL BUILDING (tour), Sacramento, California, (916) 324-0333.

CHICAGO MERCANTILE EXCHANGE, Chicago, Illinois, (312) 648-8230.

DAVEY CROCKETT BIRTHPLACE PARK, Greeneville, Tennessee, (615) 257-2061.

DEATH VALLEY NATIONAL MONUMENT, Death Valley, California, (714) 786-2331.

FRANKLIN MINT MUSEUM OF MEDALLIC ART, Franklin Center, Pennsylvania, (215) 459-6875.

HALEAKALA NATIONAL PARK, Haleakala, Hawaii, (808) 572-7749.

HAWAII VOLCANOES NATIONAL PARK, Hawaii, (808) 967-7977.

HUNTINGTON LIBRARY, San Marino, California, (818) 405-2141.

INDEPENDENCE HALL, Philadelphia, Pennsylvania, (215) 597-8974.

J. PAUL GETTY MUSEUM, Malibu, California, (213) 458-2003.

LINCOLN HOME NATIONAL HISTORIC SITE, Springfield, Illinois, (217) 492-4150.

LYNDON B. JOHNSON SPACE CENTER, Houston, Texas, (713) 483-4321.

MILLER BREWING COMPANY, Milwaukee, Wisconsin, (414) 931-2153.

MONTEZUMA NATIONAL WILDLIFE REFUGE, Seneca Falls, New York, (315) 568-5987.

MT. RUSHMORE NATIONAL MEMORIAL, Keystone, South Dakota, (605) 574-2523.

NASA VISITORS CENTER, Hampton, Viginia, (804) 722-2567.

NATIONAL HALL OF FAME FOR FAMOUS AMERICAN INDIANS, Anakarko, Oklahoma, (405) 247-6652.

NAVAL AVIATION MUSEUM, Pensacola, Florida, (904) 452-3604.

NBC STUDIO TOURS & TAPING TICKETS, Burbank, California, (818) 840-3537.

OLD U.S. MINT, San Francisco, California, (415) 974-0788.

REDWOOD NATIONAL PARK, Crescent City, California, (707) 464-6101.

SCRIPPS AQUARIUM-MUSEUM, La Jolla, California, (619) 452-6933.

TEMPLE SQUARE, MORMAN TEMPLE, THE TABERNACLE, Salt Lake City, Utah, (801) 531-2534.

THE ALAMO, San Antonio, Texas, (512) 225-1391.

TOMB OF THE UNKNOWN SOLDIER, Arlington, Virginia, (708) 683-2007.

ULYSSES S. GRANT HOME, Galena, Illinois, (815) 777-0248.

UNIVERSITY OF CALIFORNIA botanical gardens, art museum, Worth Ryder Gallery, herbarium, paleontology museum, Berkeley, California, (415) 642-5215.

U.S. COAST GUARD ACADEMY, New London, Connecticut, (203) 444-8270.

VALLEY FORGE NATIONAL HISTORICAL PARK, Valley Forge, Pennsylvania, (215) 783-7700.

WEST POINT MUSEUM, West Point, New York, (914) 938-2638.

WRIGHT BROTHERS NATIONAL MEMORIAL, Kitty Hawk, North Carolina, (919) 441-7430.

Our nation's capitol, Washington, D.C., has more than three dozen free places of interest, museums, and historical sites, including the BUREAU OF ENGRAVING AND PRINTING, the F.B.I., FORD'S THEATER AND LINCOLN MUSEUM, the KENNEDY CENTER, the LIBRARY OF CONGRESS, the NATIONAL GALLERY OF ART, the SMITHSONIAN INSTITUTION GROUP museums, the CAPITOL, the WHITE HOUSE, the NATIONAL ARCHIVES, etc. This city is like a giant candy store full of free and exciting sights. For a free booklet that describes major attractions, information on parking, neighborhoods, the Metro, theaters, etc. write: D.C. Convention and Visitors Association, Attn: Tourist Info, 1212 New York Ave. NW, Washington, D.C. 20005. There is also a free 100-page directory, the "Gold Mine Directory," that lists more than 1,700 Washington area businesses that provide discounts for people age 60 and over including hotels, inns, restaurants, entertainment facilities, shops, art galleries, bookstores, and sightseeing tours. For a copy contact The D.C. COMMITTEE TO PROMOTE WASHINGTON, 415 12th St., N.W., Suite 312, Washington, D.C. 20004.

For a complete state by state listing of free tourist attractions throughout the U.S. write for *The National Directory of Free Tourist Attractions*, *($3.95), Pilot Books, 103 Cooper St., Babylon, NY 11702.*

The following is a sampling of cultural and educational attractions that offer senior discounts:

Nature

DALLAS ZOO, Dallas, Texas. (214) 670-6825; $1 seniors ($5 regular admission).

INDIANAPOLIS ZOO, Indianapolis, Indiana. (317) 630-2001; $5 seniors ($7 regular admission).

LOS ANGELES STATE AND COUNTRY ARBORETUM, Arcadia, California. (818) 821-3222; $1.50 seniors ($3 regular admission).

LOS ANGELES ZOO, Los Angeles, California. (213) 666-4090; $5 seniors ($6 regular admission).

MILWAUKEE COUNTY ZOO, Milwaukee, Wisconsin. (414) 771-3040; $3 seniors ($4.50 regular admission).

MISSOURI BOTANICAL GARDEN, St. Louis, Missouri. (314) 577-5100; $1 seniors ($2 regular admission, free admission Wed. and Sat. 7 A.M.-noon).

MONTEREY BAY AQUARIUM, Monterey, California. (408) 648-4888; $5.75 seniors ($8 regular admission).

THE NATIONAL AQUARIUM, Washington, D.C. (202) 377-2826; $.75 seniors ($2 regular admission).

OAKLAND ZOO, Oakland, California. (415) 632-9525; $1.50 seniors ($3.50 regular admission).

PHILADELPHIA ZOO, Philadelphia, Pennsylvania. (215) 243-1100; $4.75 seniors ($5.75 regular admission).

JOHN G. SHEDD AQUARIUM, Chicago, Illinois. (312) 939-2438; $2 seniors ($3 regular admission).

THE STEINHART AQUARIUM, Golden Gate Park, San Francisco, California. (415) 221-5100; $2 seniors ($4 regular admission).

Museums

AMERICAN CRAFT MUSEUM, New York, New York. (212) 956-6047; $1.50 seniors ($3.50 regular admission).

AMERICAN MUSEUM OF NATURAL HISTORY and HAYDEN PLANETARIUM, New York, New York. (212) 769-5900; $3 seniors ($4 regular admission).

ART INSTITUTE OF CHICAGO, Chicago, Illinois. (312) 443-3600; $3 seniors suggested donation ($6 regular suggested donation, free on Tuesday).

THE B&O RAILROAD MUSEUM, Baltimore, Maryland. (301) 752-2490; $4 seniors ($5 regular admission).

BOSTON TEA PARTY SHIP AND MUSEUM, Boston, Massachusetts. (617) 338-1773; $4 seniors ($5 regular admission).

CINCINNATI ART MUSEUM, Cincinnati, Ohio. (513) 721-5204; $1.50 seniors ($3 regular admission).

DENVER ART MUSEUM, Denver, Colorado. (303) 640-2793; $1.50 seniors ($3 regular admission).

FINE ARTS MUSEUM OF SAN FRANCISCO (De Young Museum), San Francisco, California. (415) 863-3330); $2 seniors ($4 regular admission).

THE FRANK LLOYD WRIGHT HOME AND STUDIO FOUNDATION, Oak Park, Illinois. (708) 848-1976; $2 senior tour fee ($4 regular tour fee).

GENE AUTRY WESTERN HERITAGE MUSEUM, Los Angeles, California. (213)667-2000; $4 seniors ($5.50 regular admission).

GEORGE C. PAGE MUSEUM, Los Angeles, California. (213) 936-2230; $1.50 seniors ($3 regular admission).

INTERNATIONAL MUSEUM OF PHOTOGRAPHY AT GEORGE EASTMAN HOUSE, Rochester, New York. (716) 271-3361; $2.50 seniors ($3 regular admission).

THE JEWISH MUSEUM, New York, New York. (212) 860-1888; $2.50 ($4.50 regular admission).

LOS ANGELES COUNTRY MUSEUM OF ART, Los Angeles, California. (213) 857-6522; $3.50 seniors ($5 regular admission).

THE METROPOLITAN MUSEUM OF ART, New York, New York. (212) 879-5500; $2.50 suggested senior citizen admission ($5 suggested regular admission).

MONTICELLO, Charlottesville, Virginia. (804) 295-8181; $6 seniors ($7 regular admission).

MUSEUM OF CONTEMPORARY ART, Los Angeles, California, (213) 621-2766; $2 seniors ($4 regular admission).

MUSEUM OF MODERN ART, New York, New York. (212)708-9480; $4 seniors ($7 regular admission).

NATIONAL AIR AND SPACE MUSEUM, Washington, D.C., (202) 357-1686; Charge for IMAX Theater and Planetarium show, $1.75 seniors ($2.75 regular admission).

NATIONAL COWBOY HALL OF FAME, Oklahoma City, Oklahoma. (405) 478-2250; $4 seniors ($5 regular admission).

THE PAUL REVERE HOUSE, Boston, Massachusetts. (617) 523-2338; $1.50 seniors ($2 regular admission).

THE SOLOMON R. GUGGENHEIM MUSEUM, New York, New York. (212) 360-3500; (Museum closed until Fall 1991. Check for senior prices).

UNIVERSITY MUSEUM OF ARCHEOLOGY AND ANTHRO-POLOGY, Philadelphia, Pennsylvania. (215) 898-4000; $1.50 senior volunteer donation ($3 regular volunteer donation).

WHITNEY MUSEUM OF AMERICAN ART, New York, New York. (212) 570-3676; $3 seniors ($5 regular admission).

The performing arts are also popular activities where seniors get a break. From theater, symphony, and ballet to circuses and acrobatic troups, seniors can enjoy many days and nights of first-class, first-run professional performances at special discounted rates from 25 to 50 percent off regular priced tickets. In the past several years, ticket prices have risen markedly, some reaching $40 to $50 for single tickets. Most senior discounts offer significant savings, that are sometimes greater at matinees and less popular performances.

There are also "rush" tickets that go on sale the day of a performance that are often 50 percent or more off the face price. A popular theater at the Music Center in Los Angeles offers "$10 Public Rush Tickets" available 10 minutes before curtain time. That's a 75 percent savings off the regular $40 ticket price! Also, check for preview performance discounts prior to official public openings. This same theater in Los Angeles was offering the best seats in the house for $20 during the preview period. If you can get several people together, you may qualify for senior group rates with reduced prices. Some performing arts organizations even offer special "senior performances" and "senior afternoon concerts." Again, it is important to inquire with box office personnel about all the possible savings opportunities before you purchase your tickets.

BUY ME SOME PEANUTS
AND CRACKER JACKS

Football, baseball, basketball, tennis, track and field, hockey, etc., generally take place in stadiums, auditoriums, and arenas, that offer senior discounts for sports events held there during the year. The same stadium may be home to more than one team or host several independent events throughout the year. Check with the office of the teams or the public relations department at the stadium for individual and group senior discounts, year-round discount cards, or special membership opportunities. During regular playing season, there are often one or more senior citizen days. These are advertised in the local newspaper and in the team's season calendar listing special events and dates.

Individual and special sports events also offer senior citizen discounts. Recently the Security Pacific Senior Golf Classic held yearly in Los Angeles offered $5 admission tickets for folks over 50. (Regular prices ranged from $8 to $15.)

CHAPTER 2

SPORTS, FITNESS, AND EXERCISE FOR SENIORS

As we move through the 1990s, the continuing emphasis on fitness and exercise will affect us all. This is especially true for seniors, as local, state, and national programs continue to thrive with the increase in participation by this age group. Pick up any magazine or newspaper targeted for seniors and you will find numerous opportunities to engage in healthful exercise programs and sports activities. Exercise is not only accepted, but it is strongly encouraged by every major medical association and organization for healthy seniors who want to live longer, fuller lives. In fact, it is nearly impossible to find a sport today that is not being enjoyed by older adults.

Along with the healthful benefits of participating in sports is the added benefit that most sports, exercise, and fitness programs can be enjoyed at substantially reduced prices. In fact, many charges are completely waived simply because you are a senior. Imagine spending a glorious day on the ski slopes for absolutely free, while others have spent up to $40 for a one-day lift ticket!

CALLING ALL ATHLETES

The U.S. National Senior Sports (formerly known as the U.S. National Senior Olympics) have been held every two years since they began at Washington University in St. Louis in 1987. In order to compete, an athlete must be 55 years or older, and must qualify at a local or state competition sanctioned by the U.S. National Senior Sports Organization (USNSO).

There are more than 500 separate events in archery, badminton, half-court basketball, bicycling, bowling, track and field, golf, horse-shoes, racewalking, 5K and 10K road races, shuffleboard, softball, swimming, table tennis, tennis, volleyball, and the triathlon. Competitions are organized for men and women and are separated into age categories. For additional information on qualification requirements and schedules of qualifying games, contact: U.S. National Senior Sports Organization, 14323 S. Outer Forty Rd., Suite N300, Chesterfield, MO 63017 (314) 878-4900.

STATE COMPETITIONS

Several states hold their own senior games, some alternating seasons similar to the summer and winter Olympics. The games often take place at local college or state university campuses. Athletes competing in these games go on to participate in the U.S. National Senior Sports Classic. In addition to the states listed below, there are programs sponsored by county, city, and local agencies which participate in the national program. Some state parks and recreation departments are also involved in senior competitions affiliated with the national games.

CALIFORNIA Senior Olympics are held annually in Palm Springs. Contact: California Senior Olympics, 550 North Palm Canyon Drive, Palm Springs, CA 92262. There is also a Northern California Senior Olympics and a San Diego Senior Olympics.

COLORADO hosts the Rocky Mountain Senior Games twice a year, in summer and winter. Contact: Rocky Mountain Senior Games, 2604 S. Pennsylvania, Denver, CO 80210.

CONNECTICUT Senior Olympics include physical fitness activities and a health fair. Contact: Connecticut Senior Olympics, Harvey Hubbell Gymnasium, University of Bridgeport, Bridgeport, CT 06601.

FLORIDA's Golden Age Games are held in Sanford annually in November. Contact: The Greater Sanford Chamber of Commerce, P.O. Drawer CC, Sanford, FL 32772.

MICHIGAN Senior Olympics are a one day event held in August in Farmington Hills. Contact the Michigan Senior Olympics, O.P.C., 312 Woodward, Rochester, MI 48063.

In MISSOURI the St. Louis Senior Olympics are held over four days. Contact: Senior Olympics, JCAA, 2 Millstone Campus, St. Louis, MO 63146.

MONTANA's Big Sky Games are held in July in Billings. Contact: The Big Sky Games, P.O. Box 2318, Billings, MT 59101.

The NEW YORK Senior Games are held in the spring and are open to state residents up to 80+. Contact: New York Senior Games, State Parks, Agency I, 12th Fl., Albany, NY 12238.

NORTH CAROLINA holds local games throughout the state. Winners compete in the state finals in Raleigh. Contact: North Carolina Senior Games, P.O. Box 33590, Raleigh, NC 27606.

PENNSYLVANIA Senior Games are a four-day event held at a university campus. Contact: Pennsylvania Senior Games, 231 State St., Harrisburg, PA 17101.

VERMONT holds the Green Mountain Senior Games in early fall in Poultney, Vermont. Contact: Green Mountain Senior Games, P.O. Box 1660, Station A, Rutland, VT 05701.

VIRGINIA holds its Golden Olympics in the spring at Lynchburg College. Contact the Golden Olympics, P.O. Box 2774, Lunchburg, VA 24501.

In WASHINGTON the Seattle Senior Sports Festival is a Regional Qualifying Event for the national games. Contact: Senior Sports Festival, 100 Dexter Ave., North, Seattle, WA 98109-51909.

Senior Sports competitions are also held in Alabama, Arizona, Arkansas, Georgia, Idaho, Illinois, Indiana, Iowa, Kansas, Kentucky, Louisiana, Maine, Maryland, Minnesota, Mississippi, Nebraska, Nevada, New Hampshire, New Jersey, New Mexico, Ohio, Oklahoma, Rhode Island, South Carolina, South Dakota, Tennessee, Texas, D.C., Wisconsin and Wyoming.

Since 1987 Huntsman Chemicals has sponsored the *WORLD SENIOR GAMES* for senior athletes 50 and above each October in Utah. Senior athletes from all parts of the world are invited to participate in events including golf, swimming, bicycling, tennis, racewalking, track and field, softball, bowling and racquetball. For information write:

Huntsman Chemical's World Senior Games, 1604 Walker Center St., Lake City, Utah 84111.

* * * * *

The UNITED STATES SENIOR ATHLETIC GAMES are also patterned after the Olympics and are open to all seniors 50 and over. The games, which have been held yearly since 1980, take place in Florida over a period of one week. There are 10 sports categories, along with special events, entertainment programs and special sports competitions. A reasonable fee of $15 for participants includes all events. For more information contact: United States Senior Athletic Games, 200 Castlewood Drive, North Palm Beach, FL 33408.

THE NATIONAL SENIOR SPORTS ASSOCIATION

THE NATIONAL SENIOR SPORTS ASSOCIATION is a nonprofit organization that assists active people over 50 in their pursuit of physical and emotional health through active sports participation. The NSSA organizes tournaments (competitive as well as recreational) in tennis, bowling, golf, skiing, and fishing at resorts around the country. They also organize sports-oriented vacations with special group rates. Members receive discounts on a variety of sports equipment and related products, information on national and international sports-related trips, a monthly newsletter, the opportunity to participate in a vacation home exchange program, and names and addresses of members in other locations. For complete information on the NSSA, write them at: NSSA, 10560 Main St., Ste. 205A, Fairfax, VA 22030, (703) 385-7540.

TENNIS—THE SPORT FOR A LIFETIME

Senior tennis is a thriving and popular sport. There are senior tournaments and competitions held at every level of play. Check with your local parks and recreation department, health or tennis club for information on instruction and tournaments. Also county tennis associations sponsor tournament play for seniors. If your local park or community center doesn't have any organized program, the UNITED STATES TENNIS ASSOCIATION has compiled a kit that shows how to launch teams of players of the same level of play. You can get the kit by sending $6.50 to: Publications, USTA Center for Education and Recreational Tennis, 707 Alexander Road, Princeton, NJ 08540. Ask for the Recreational Senior Tennis League kit.

The USTA holds Senior National Championships each year at tennis facilities throughout the country. There are divisions for men's and women's singles and doubles, from age 30 through 85, Father-Son Doubles, and Mother-Daughter Doubles. Write the USTA at 1212 Avenue of the Americas, New York, NY 10036, for their Senior National Championship brochure, which includes dates of play, locations, requirements, fees, and a section on health notes. The USTA also publishes a "Senior Tennis Directory" for $6.50. You can write for this guide and a complete list of current USTA Tennis Publications at: USTA, Publications Department, 707 Alexander Road, Princeton, New Jersey 08540.

The USTA/VOLVO TENNIS LEAGUE provides a framework for team competition at local levels, culminating in playoffs in which teams travel outside their local area playing a series of championships at district, sectional and national levels. The league offers senior competition in every USTA section of the United States except the Carribean.

RUN FOR YOUR LIFE

The 50-PLUS RUNNERS ASSOCIATION promotes exchange of information between the growing numbers of over-50 runners. Formed by researchers from Stanford University the group also encourages studies of the effects and impact of running on different aspects of life. Members receive an excellent quarterly newsletter, *Fifty-Plus Bulletin,* and participate in continuing studies and surveys. A voluntary contribution of $20 is requested. For information contact: Fifty-Plus Runners Association, P.O. Box D, Stanford, CA 94309.

THE ROAD RUNNERS CLUB OF AMERICA has over 450 local affiliates throughout the country. The popular, "Run For Your Life" program, a physical fitness program, originated with this group. For brochures and information on their programs and services contact: Road Runners Club of America, 629 South Washington Street, Alexandria, VA 22314.

Another organization that promotes running is the AMERICAN RUNNING AND FITNESS ASSOCIATION, 2001 S. Street, N.W., Suite 540, Washington, D.C. 20001. Write them for information on their programs.

TAKE YOURSELF OUT TO THE BALL GAME

Baseball is another popular senior sport enjoyed by over 200,000 people. THE NATIONAL ASSOCIATION OF SENIOR CITIZENS SOFTBALL promotes international interest in the game and sponsors teams throughout the country. Members receive a quarterly newsletter and have the opportunity of playing in a yearly national tournament and exhibition games and tournaments around the world. For information write: National Association of Senior Citizen Softball, Box 1085, Mt. Clemens, MI 48046.

If you are not a participator, but love baseball, many of the major and minor league team baseball teams offer senior discount days and reduced priced tickets for clubs. Check with the group ticket office of your local baseball team for these special offers.

THE AMATEUR SOFTBALL ASSOCIATION provides information on local leagues and how to start up a softball league. They also coordinate tournaments for 55+ league players. Contact them at: Amateur Softball Association, 2801 Northeast 50th Street, Oklahoma City, OK 73111.

IF YOU'RE ON A ROLL, BOWL

Bowling is another great sport for seniors and has grown tremendously over the past decade. Senior leagues and tournaments are very popular, and most bowling alleys reduce game fees for both individuals and groups. Also, since bowling alleys are usually less crowded during the daytime hours, this is one of the best times for senior bowling. THE AMERICAN BOWLING CONGRESS (ABC, Bowling Headquarters, 5301 South 76th Street, Greendale, WI 53129) will send you information on bowling for older adults and where there are leagues in your area.

If your local bowling alley is a member of the American Bowling Congress or WOMEN'S INTERNATIONAL BOWLING CONGRESS, you can ask them to send you the 12-part "Bowling for Seniors" packet, which contains ideas on starting leagues, scoring, tournaments, bowling film rentals, and other ideas on developing an active senior program. Or contact your neighborhood bowling center about joining their senior leagues.

WALK FOR HEALTH

Probably the fastest growing active sport for older adults today is walking. The number of exercise walkers 55+ has more than doubled in recent years, from approximately 8.6 million in 1985 to more than 20 million. Not only is walking good for the heart, but it has also been established that it's good for the bones as well. A recent study found that through a regular schedule of walking, jogging, or climbing stairs, men and women can build stronger bones and help prevent osteoporosis, a disease prevalent in older adults, especially women. Women who exercise regularly can actually increase bone mass in the spine, helping give bones strength and resistance to fracture. The study also found that the typical serious walker is a 53-year old woman who walks an average of 15 miles a week.

Walking programs, clinics, and clubs can be found in almost every town and city in the country. Indoor shopping malls have become popular places to walk (after a walk around the block or the park) because of their safe environment and availability year-round, regardless of weather conditions. In addition, some organized clubs sponsor lectures on a wide range of health topics given by physicians and health professionals. From Walk-A-Dillies to Senior Strutters, there are community groups for walking in your area. Check with local senior citizen groups, "senior" newspapers, community centers and medical facilities to locate a walking club or program in your area.

THE WALKERS CLUB OF AMERICA, a national organization that promotes fitness through walking, will send you a free list of walking clinics and clubs by enclosing a SASE (self-addressed stamped envelope) to: The Walkers Club of America, Box M, Livingston Manor, NY 12758. You can also contact the NATIONAL ASSOCIATION OF MALL

WALKERS, P.O. Box 191, Hermann, MO 65041, or Walkways Center, 1400 16th Street, N.W., Washington, D.C. 20036, for information on their organizations.

THE ROCKPORT WALKING INSTITUTE offers a free walking bro-chure, "The Rockport Guide to Fitness Walking." The brochure contains a self-administered fitness assessment and a 20-week walking program designed for various fitness levels and ages. Enclose a $.45 SASE to: The Rockport Walking Institute, P.O. Box 480, Marlboro, MA 01752.

For those who would like to learn more about the sport of racewalking, send a SASE to Bruce Douglass, Racewalking Chairman, The Athletics Congress, P.O. Box 120, Indianapolis, IN 46206. They will send back a free directory of racewalking clubs and information on the sport.

If you want to commit serious outside time to walking, you can go to the SPARTA HEALTH SPA AND FITNESS CENTER in the Catskill Forest Preserve, a 100-acre camp for walkers. For information write: Sparta Health Spa, Box M, Livingston Manor, NY 12758.

Finally, there are several good books and pamphlets available in your bookstore or library on walking including:

The Rockport Walking Program, by James Rippe, M.D. and Ann Ward, Ph.D., published by Prentice-Hall.

Fitness Walking for Women, by Anne Kashiwa and James Rippe, M.D., Putnam Publishing Group.

Racewalk to Fitness, by Howard Jacobson, available through Walkers Club of America Press (see address above).

THE CLASSIC GAME OF GOLF

Although seniors have been aware of it for decades, the game of golf has recently enjoyed an international resurgence, in part due to the tremendous popularity it has found among the Japanese, who have embraced the sport with a passion. Most public and many private golf courses will give a discount on greens fees for seniors over 65.

THE GOLF CARD which costs $75 a year for single membership and $120 for a couple, was designed especially with seniors in mind. It entitles members to play two free rounds of 18-hole golf at nearly 1,650 member golf courses around the world. As a Golf Card bearer, you also receive Golf Traveler magazine, a directory and guide to member courses and resorts participating in the program, as well as discounts on golf vacation packages at nearly 400 member resorts.

There is no minimum age requirement to join the program, however the average age for members is 61. For more information write: The Golf Card, Dept. NC, 1137 E. 2100 South, P.O. Box 526439, Salt Lake City, UT 84152. Or call (800) 453-4260.

THE PACIFIC AMATEUR GOLF ASSOCIATION (PAGA) offers golfing tours that also include sightseeing. They are called "golferama carousels" because you can take all or part of the tours. There are also activities for the nongolfing partners while the golfers are playing. Tours include the Pacific Northwest North, Pacific Northwest South, Colorful Colorado, Rockies to Remember, New Mexico, and Eastern Canada. Seniors receive a discount on tour packages. For more information write: PAGA, 426 E. Dartmouth Road, Burbank, CA 91504.

Many senior golf competitions and tournaments are held by public and private organizations and clubs throughout the year. Charities have found that sponsoring senior golf tournaments is a great way to raise funds and enlist older adults in a healthy, fun activity. Many regular tournaments advertise special senior discounts for daily or multi-day passes. For instance, daily ground passes for the week-long Los Angeles Open Golf Tournament cost $15 per day. Senior passes are $10 per day, adding up to some good savings if you plan to attend several days. Check with public golf courses, Departments of Parks and Recreation, and senior publications for their local activities, tournaments, and senior discounts.

YOU'RE NEVER TOO OLD TO SKI

Believe it or not, skiing is a very popular sport among older adults, and there are several clubs and discounts specifically targeted for this age group. For those taking up the sport for the first time, or for veteran skiers who have been schussing down the slopes for decades, with great deals available for seniors, this may be the best time of all to enjoy this exciting sport.

THE OVER THE HILL GANG originated with a group of older skiers looking for other older skiers to ski with. They are now an international skiing group whose members get discounts on lifts, rentals, group guides, ski clinics, and group lessons. They offer a yearly Senior Ski Week that takes place at a ski resort in the Rockies or Europe and week-vacation packages at several resorts around Lake Tahoe, California. Local Gang groups also organize ski trips with their own members or meet to ski weekly at local ski resorts. For information on membership write: Over the Hill Gang International, 13791 E. Rice Pl, Aurora, CO 80015, or call (303) 699-6404.

If you can prove you are over 70, you can join the 70+ SKI CLUB which boasts over 3,000 members. One of the original purposes of this group was to make skiing more affordable for older adults on fixed or limited retirement incomes. Club members meet as a group every year for an annual meeting and participate in the 70+ Ski Races at Hunter Mountain in the Catskills. Cost of a lifetime membership is $5, and includes a newsletter and list of ski areas across the country offering free or discounted skiing for seniors. For information write: 70+ Ski Club, 104 Eastside Drive, Ballston Lake, NY 12019.

If you ski in the east, there are several ski clubs organized for older adults. These include:

THE BROMLEY SENIOR SKIERS CLUB, Bromley Mountain, Box 1130, Manchester Center, VT 05255.

MOUNT SNOW SENIORSKI, Mt. Snow, VT 05356.

STRATTON SENIOR SKIERS ASSOCIATION, c/o Vermont Ski Areas Association, Box 368, Montpelier, VT 05602.

WATERVILLE VALLEY SILVER STREAKS, Stratton Senior Skiers, Stratton Mountain, VT 05155.

Ski resorts throughout the country offer older adults discounts on tickets, rentals, and other amenities. Many discounts range from 50 percent off lift tickets to free tickets and seasons passes for adults over 55. For example, 46 ski areas or resorts in Michigan offer free downhill or cross-country skiing to people over 55. If you are thinking of taking a ski vacation, check the discounts on vacation packages at hotels and ski lodges associated with the ski area's operators. Always ask about the senior discounts before purchasing daily lift tickets or tickets included with tours and vacation packages.

Even if you don't ski, how about taking the grandchildren on a ski vacation, sharing in the fun and action, and perhaps taking a lesson as well? Weekdays are often slow times at ski resorts, and many offer midweek family plans at greatly reduced rates, often including free lodging (and sometimes lift passes) for the kids.

CROSS-COUNTRY SKIING

Cross-country skiing is another popular form of exercise that provides an excellent aerobic workout, yet takes it easy on the joints. More than 6.5 million Americans enjoy this sport, which not only costs considerably less than downhill skiing, but also avoids annoying waits in long lift lines. Although many people believe that, "If you can walk, you can cross-country ski," it's not as simple as that. The CROSS COUNTRY SKI AREAS ASSOCIATION recommends that everyone take a lesson or two to become familiar with the equipment and techniques. The CCSAA has a $2 directory called "Destinations" that lists more than 200 cross-country ski areas, many of which offer discounts for seniors. To order write: Cross Country Ski Areas Association, 259 Bolton Road, Winchester, NH 03470.

For serious cross-country skiers, the WORLD MASTERS CROSS-COUNTRY SKI ASSOCIATION sponsors yearly international races. Participants must be over 30, and events are separated into five-year age groups up to 75+. For information contact: World Masters Cross-Country Ski Association USA, 332 Iowa Avenue, P.O. Box 718, Hayward, WI 54843.

In addition to asking for senior discounts at the more than 800 cross-country ski areas around the country, there are a variety of special packages offered by travel companies. A few include: The ASPEN SKIING COMPANY'S programs for skiers over 50 called The Fit for Life 50/Plus program. Call (800) 952-1515 for details; OUTDOOR VACATIONS FOR WOMEN OVER 40 offers cross-country ski clinics, weekend and longer packages for women who like adventurous outdoor vacations. Write: Women Over 40, P.O. Box 200, Groton, MA 01450; ELDERHOSTEL combines its educational programs with low-cost cross-country ski vacations near its educational sites. For information write: Elderhostel, 80 Boylston St., Suite 400, Boston, MA 02116; and WATERVILLE VALLEY, a New Hampshire ski area, has a cross-country ski package, the Old-Fashioned Winter Getaway, for skiers over 55. This is a complete weekend package including most meals, wine and cheese party, cross-country classes, a sleigh ride, morning stretch classes, and a guided ski tour with picnic lunch. Call the Waterville Valley Lodging Bureau at (800) 258-8988.

DANCING

Dancing is by far the most popular social exercise enjoyed by older adults. It is fun, nonstressing, friendly, and good for you. Look in the activities section of your local newspaper or "senior" newspaper and you will most likely find a senior dance event happening that same week. One Southern California senior citizen newspaper listed no fewer than 12 dance events. Weekly dances and dance classes are held at recreation centers, senior clubs, churches, and community centers.

STAY IN SHAPE WITH SWIMMING

Swimming is often recommended for people with arthritis and back or leg injuries. Some fitness experts consider it the healthiest and best overall sport and all-around conditioner. In addition, swimming is one of the most injury-free sports because there is less stress on the joints and muscle system. It is also an inexpensive sport that does not require a lot of special equipment or training.

Swimming is so good for you, in fact, it has been the most popular participation sport in the United States for the past four years. For information on pool locations, lap times and classes contact your health club, YMCA, YWCA, or city Parks and Recreation Department.

VOLKSSPORTING

The AMERICAN VOLKSSPORT ASSOCIATION is a nonprofit, volunteer organization whose goal is to promote physical fitness and good health by encouraging all people, regardless of age, to exercise in noncompetitive, stress-free programs. Volkssports are organized, noncompetitive walking, swimming, bicycling and cross-country skiing events. Each event has a premarked scenic trail and/or measured distance designed to appeal to all ages. There are even special provisions for the handicapped to participate in most events. Participation is free of charge.

Volkssporting is an especially beneficial opportunity for seniors who cannot, should not, or simply don't want to exercise in timed or competitive events. Seniors have an equal chance to participate in programs of exercise and fun where no special training or equipment is required and at the same time is safe. Participants in the Lifesports program choose the sport(s), the distance(s), and the pace.

The American Volkssport Association has over 600 member clubs chartered in 49 states. The AVA publishes *The American Wanderer*, a bimonthly newsletter of Volkssporting news, calendar of events, AVA club list, and other information. For information write: American Volkssport Association, Suite 203, Phoenix Square, 1001 Pat Booker Road, Universal City, TX 78148.

NONSTRESS EXERCISE

Not everyone is able to join in the sports and activities described in these last few pages. However, almost everyone can exercise in some way. Arthritis, one of the most common villains in the battle against growing older, limits millions from participating in the more vigorous, active sports. Range-of-motion exercises (for flexibility and range of movement), stretching, and strength-building programs are enthusiastically supported by the medical community for those having any of the more than 100 different rheumatic disorders.

THE ARTHRITIS FOUNDATION has over 70 chapters throughout the country that offer free educational courses, exercise programs, and support resources. They also publish an exercise brochure filled with safety tips and examples of safe, range-of-motion exercises. For information contact: The Arthritis Foundation, P.O. Box 19000, Atlanta, GA 30326.

THE AMERICAN PHYSICAL THERAPY ASSOCIATION will send you a free guide sheet with stretching tips to avoid some of the stiffness and minor pain associated with exercise and sports. Send for "Guidelines for Greater Enjoyment of an Active Life," Public Relations Dept., American Physical Therapy Association, 1111 No. Fairfax St., Alexandria, VA 22314.

"THE FITNESS CHALLENGE ...IN LATER YEARS" is a guide outlining an exercise program for maintaining youthful health and energy and suggests ways of enhancing the enjoyment of leisure. For a copy write: U.S. Dept. of Health and Human Services, Commissioner on Aging, 200 Independence Ave. SW, Washington, D.C. 20201.

Once you've finished all that terrific exercise that's keeping you fit and healthy, you might want a nice soothing massage to help relax those muscles you've worked so hard. THE AMERICAN MASSAGE THERAPY ASSOCIATION will send you a free booklet, "A Guide to Massage Therapy in America." Write them at AMTA, 1130 W. North Shore Ave., Chicago, IL 60626.

BUSINESS AND EXERCISE

The Senior Healthtrac Program by Blue Shield of California, was the first preventive/positive health care program developed and operated by an insurance company. The program is intended to reduce the risks of illness related to chronic disease and help lower hospital and medical costs through decreased dependency on health care services. Policyholders over age 65 participating in the program are supplied with educational materials containing nutritional guidelines, exercise programs, and healthful lifestyle changes. In addition, Healthtrac has a continuing program of health educational materials to assist seniors in making needed health improvements. A recent study among retirees at high risk for medical problems has shown that the numerous health benefits gained by participants can actually save individuals as much as $4,500 a year in health costs.

In line with the Healthtrac program, many companies encourage older workers and retirees to participate in a variety of self-directed and group exercise programs. The Adolph Coors Company's "Senior Aerobics" class is geared toward gentler stretching exercises. John Hancock's Walkers Club has been a successful means to promote participation of older workers, while other recreational activities appealing to older adults (such as square dancing at Goodyear Tire) have also been implemented. The Campbell Soup Company encourages older employees and retirees to use their fitness center and join in flexibility exercise classes, while Texas Instruments has inaugurated "Fit to be

50" classes and provides advice on nutrition and dealing with stress. In the end, by helping senior employees and retirees lead healthier lives, these companies are actively working to reduce their enormous health cost liabilities among this age group.

CHAPTER 3

SERIOUS SHOPPING AND SAVINGS

Mature adults are a loyal group when it comes to shopping and choosing products and services. Smart retailers and companies in the business of serving the public know that mature people want quality and service they can depend on, and will reward those who satisfy their needs by coming back again and again.

Two of the nation's largest retailers have discount programs specifically targeted to seniors, SEARS and MONTGOMERY WARD. Sears' program, Mature Outlook, offers among other benefits, significant discounts in the form of coupons that can be used for a variety of products and services. Montgomery Ward has a Y.E.S. (Years of Extra Savings) Club. Members get 10 percent off any merchandise purchased in Montgomery Ward stores every Tuesday. There is also a 10 percent discount every day off any of Montgomery Ward's auto services.

Other major chain stores that offer senior citizen discounts include:

AMES DEPARTMENT STORES. Over 455 locations in New England. Offers 10 percent senior citizen discount on unadvertised merchandise. Individual stores have "Senior Discount Day."

FAMILY DOLLAR STORES. More than 1,600 stores in 27 states and Washington, D.C. Offers 10 percent senior citizen Tuesday discount on all merchandise.

WALDENBOOKS. More than 1,000 stores throughout the country. The "Preferred Reader Program" entitles members to 10 percent discount on all books and accessories (including items on sale). There is a onetime $5 membership fee for those 60 years or older.

Senior citizen newspapers often carry advertising by local establishments for discounts of at least 10 percent. Some discounts are good only on certain days of the week or are offered on a "limited time only" basis. In most cases you need to ask for the discount at the time of purchase or service. Here are some recent examples of discounts:

- 10 percent off toys, games, and hobbies at regional chain of toy stores.

- 15 percent on any purchase, regular or sale, for one day at a popular chain department store.

- Senior citizen discount coupons available from a local taxi company.

- Senior citizen discounts from a distributor of medical, burglary, and fire alarms and security systems.

- 10 percent senior citizen discount for all automotive service repairs from a tire and brake service garage.

- 10 percent discount to seniors over 50 on all orders from a collectibles mail order catalog.

- Senior citizen coupon worth $1 off the cost of a car wash.

- 10 percent senior citizen discount on television repair service.

- 10 percent senior citizen discount on window washing.

- 10 percent senior citizen discount on veterinarian services.

- 20 percent senior citizen discount on medical services of a general practitioner.

- 15 to 25 percent senior citizen discount on dental services.

- 15 percent senior citizen discount on the services of an electrician and 10 percent off the cost of services of a handyman.

- Senior discount offered on house painting, carpentry, and concrete and block work.

- 41 percent senior citizen discount on regular price acrylic yarn from super yarn mart.

If you want to take advantage of self-service prices at gas stations, but have a problem doing it yourself (pumping gas can be hard on stiff joints and limbs), individual station owners are often sympathetic to the less agile older citizen's plight. Speak with the manager or owner about arranging a time to come in for gas when business is usually slow. They will help you fill up at the self-service tank when they are not busy with other customers. Avoid gas station-convenience store combos or high-volume gas stations. Some operate with only one or two cashiers who are unable to leave their posts to help customers.

State senior citizen discount programs include businesses offering senior discounts (in addition to the discounts seniors receive at state parks, campgrounds, fishing areas, historic sites, etc.). A member of the program can use his or her membership card to obtain discounts at establishments participating in the senior discount program. In California, participants advertising in the Yellow Pages of the phone directory display a special symbol in their ads to notify consumers that they belong to the program. Check with your state's Office/Department on Aging for a list of businesses in the senior citizen discount program.

CHAPTER 4

"TIME OF YOUR LIFE" TRAVEL

Welcome to the world of senior travel! Today's mature adults have more freedom to travel without the restrictions and responsibilities of supporting children, busy households, complicated schedules, and building careers. Traveling can be a learning experience, an adventure, a much-deserved chance to relax, a physical challenge, or whatever you dream it to be. After waiting this many years, you can be flexible and travel wherever you want, as long as you want, and whenever you want. This translates into lots of savings because, in addition to year-round senior discounts, you can make your travel plans during those times when airline, hotel, car rental, cruise, etc., prices are at their lowest. By using the methods outlined in this chapter, you can save as much as 85 percent on fares and accommodations. Exotic island winter trips, distant European holidays, and cross-country visits to see the grandchildren are just a few of the possibilities. The "trip of a lifetime" can come more than once for mature adults who take advantage of the opportunities available to them.

Travel is the number one desire and activity of the 50+ age group. In fact, 80 percent of all pleasure travel is by individuals over 50. In addition, they take more trips per year, travel longer distances, and spend more time away from home than any other age group. What this means to the travel industry is that seniors spend more money, on the whole, than anyone else: more than $51 million yearly on travel, and by the year 1995, that figure will rise to $56 million.

As a result, the travel industry has vigorously courted the mature adult market by creating numerous discount programs, tours, packages, etc., just for them. Travel agents, airlines, cruise lines, hotels, and other travel businesses know mature adults are free to travel at off-peak times or whenever they desire a change of scenery. They also know that this age group includes shrewd, experienced travelers who look for the best deals to the best places.

The travel industry has also reduced the burden of planning vacations by creating an array of choices and ways to travel, thus relieving seniors of the tedious details of "do it yourself" vacations. Even if you are an experienced traveler, planning a trip can become quite complicated. Since deregulation, there are many excellent, money saving deals available, but rates, fares, and privileges can change at a moments notice. There is such a variety of fares and accommodations, it's difficult to know if you are really getting the most for your money. It's important to be as thorough as possible in checking out current prices.

TRAVELING FOR FREE

There are several ways mature adults can take advantage of the little-known "tricks of the trade" within the travel industry to earn free travel. Most free travel requires no special skills, credentials, or contacts. And it can be as luxurious and pleasurable as the most expensive paid vacation. Consider the following if you want to see the world and do it at somebody else's expense:

- Become a tour escort for a travel agency that operate tours; a senior citizen center or clubs with tour programs; or a professional tour operator. Tour operators are always looking for interesting people to lead their tours, especially during the summer tourist season. You will act as tour leader/manager for the group with all your expenses paid. If you are fluent in one or more languages, your services will be especially desirable for tours to foreign countries.

- Organize your own tour or group. If you can enlist enough people, you can get a whole trip, long or short, for free. Some travel agencies recruit teachers who receive a free trip if they bring six students. With 12 students, your spouse can join you for free. Traveling free as a teacher is a very popular way to visit places that would otherwise be financially prohibitive.

- Work for a travel agency. By becoming trained as a travel agent you can qualify for large travel discounts and free travel. Travel agents can often work part-time or from home and still receive the same benefits as full-time counselors.

- Organize a "special interest" tour. If you are a wine aficionado, you might organize a trip to the French wine country; or put together a group from your church for a religious pilgrimage to a Holy Land; or travel to Vienna and Salzburg with other opera buffs. Special-interest trips focus on everything from golf, tennis, and bicycling to photography, archaeology, history, theater, music, and gourmet food. A good travel agent can create a tour around your group's common interest. And by organizing and providing the travelers, you will earn a free trip.

- Travel free as a travel writer. If you like to travel and have a flair for writing, you have a good chance of paying for your travels by selling your experiences, short stories, photos, etc., to publications and newspapers that are looking for a new point of view about a different place. Nearly every mature adult publication and dozens of consumer magazines and newspapers can use feature stories, photo spreads and columns on travel, since it is one of the most popular topics of interest to readers.

- Become an air courier. An air courier is someone who accompanies freight (usually small parcels and envelopes filled with documents) which has been checked as baggage on a flight. In the case of foreign flights, the package arrives with the courier and is processed through customs immediately along with the courier's other bags rather than remaining in a warehouse waiting customs clearance. Courier companies offer assignments to the general public in exchange for free or deeply discounted tickets (70 percent or more). The key to becoming a courier is being flexible and able to travel light and within the time table of the courier firm. Courier firms want their representatives to maintain a well-dressed, respectable image and welcome responsible mature people they can rely on.

- Buy a new automobile overseas. Several European delivery specialists will pay your round-trip airfare if you buy an automobile from them and pick it up over there. They also arrange all necessary customs and vehicle inspections once the car arrives in the United States. You can save from $4,000 to $7,000 on a new Jaguar, BMW, Mercedes, Volvo, Saab, Porsche, Audi, Volkswagon, etc., by arranging European delivery.

- Become a lecturer, performer, or organizer aboard a cruise ship. You can cruise free as an expert on a specific subject, business, or other interesting field. Historians, anthropologists, naturalists, former athletes, coaches, musicians, cosmetologists, writers, entertainers, retired executives, CEOs, teachers, etc. are always in high demand to provide guests with an entertaining and interesting array of information and activities. Your job would be to present a series of lectures, organize activities, etc., and be available for informal demonstrations and discussions. In return you receive an all expenses paid cruise.

- A great way to *stretch* your travel dollars is to participate in a home exchange program. There are several books, clubs and exchange services that list thousands of homes around the world whose owners offer club members a free stay for a week or more. THE INTERNATIONAL HOME EXCHANGE SERVICE publishes three directories a year with more than 7,000 listings and details on how to set up an exchange. More than 80 percent of the listings are from outside the United States, ranging as far as Brazil, Nepal, Australia, and Zimbabwe, but most exchange homes abroad are in Europe. Subscriptions are $55 per year. For information contact BOOK PASSAGE, (800) 321-9785 or INTERNATIONAL HOME EXCHANGE SERVICE, (415) 956-1011.

- If you want to learn all about home exchanges and how they work, *Swap and Go*, by Arthur Frommer and co-authors Albert and Verna Beerbower (Englewood Cliffs, NJ: Prentice Hall) explains everything there is to know about these programs and what you need to set up your own home for exchange. There is also a listing of home exchange agencies. The book is $10.95 and can be ordered through Book Passage, (800) 321-9785.

- Finally, if you like the idea of a free place to stay, consider becoming a professional house-sitter. This is one way to enjoy beautifully furnished (sometimes including maid-service) homes and mansions for free. Most people would rather not abandon their pets to a strange kennel or leave their houses vacant while they travel. A professional house-sitter can spend nearly all year helping different folks out by watching their houses and pets, usually getting paid for it. Free house-sitting works in the opposite way as well. People who own expensive vacation and resort homes often visit these homes only once or twice a year. They also want the peace of mind of having their homes watched over and cared for while they are not there. When they arrive for their vacation, you can visit friends or relatives while they are vacationing in "your" home. How does year-round living in Key West, Florida; Kannapali Beach, Maui; Aspen, Colorado or Malibu, California sound? Many people have homes in the Bahamas, Mexico and other foreign countries that they prefer to be lived in year-round.

• Another way to live and travel-around for free is by house-sitting for homes that are for sale. Houses built for "spec" and model homes especially are perfect for house-sitting. Higher priced homes often stay on the market for several months at a time. Meanwhile, you are enjoying a brand new home. Older homes up for sale are often left empty because their owners have already moved into new homes. Fine homes with swimming pools, tennis courts and lush gardens need someone to watch over them so vandals don't take advantage of their being empty for long periods of time.

PLANNING TRIPS AND USING TRAVEL AGENCIES

The simplest and best place to start planning a trip is with a professional travel agency. (Choose one that is a member of the American Society of Travel Agents [ASTA].) Most services and counseling provided by travel agents is free of charge. Agents make their money from commissions paid by airlines or other travel businesses.

You can choose a travel agency that specializes in a particular type of travel or travel to a specific geographic area. There are agencies that specialize in cruises, general pleasure travel, or business travel. Some handle groups and tours while others work only with individual travelers.

There are travel agents who book trips mainly to Mexico, South America, or Europe.

Here are some questions to ask yourself when choosing a travel agent:

- Are your personal travel requests considered by the agent (such as first- or ground-floor accommodations, in-room amenities, smoking or nonsmoking seats and hotel rooms, bellman to carry heavy luggage)?

- When discussing budgets, are you asked about your flexibility in making travel arrangements?

- Are you asked about health concerns?

- Will your travel agent follow through on your behalf, especially if a problem arises during you trip?

If the answers to these questions are "yes," then you have found a good agency for your travel plans.

Some travel agencies have their customers fill out "personal profile" forms, which aid them in choosing the most appropriate arrangements. If your agency doesn't have such a form, you can help them by making a list of the kinds of activities, recreation, and accommodations you prefer. Also make a rough budget of what you expect to spend and save. If you hate traveling in groups or you don't want to spend more than $40 for dinner, or you prefer to shop rather than sightsee, list those desires as well. Take travel brochures from the agency to help you. Travel agents can advance-book everything from hotel reservations and transportation, to theater tickets and dinner reservations. Working closely with them will assure you of a smooth-running, well-planned trip.

Should you plan your trip yourself? Since fares and rates sometimes change daily, a travel agency's sophisticated computer systems linked to thousands of current prices, gives them the advantage by having this information at their fingertips. If you are planning a complex trip including many stops, we suggest using a professional travel agent. A recent survey of New York City travel agents showed that prices quoted for the lowest air fare to other cities varied more than 50 percent. Some travel agents quote the first price they see and don't bother to find out about the bargains. This shows how important it is to establish a working relationship with a single travel agent who will be more inclined to spend time on your travel needs. Ask your friends, family and associates to recommend a good agent, or contact one of the sources below to help in your search:

AMERICAN SOCIETY OF TRAVEL AGENTS (ASTA)
World Headquarters
1101 King Street
Alexandria, VA 22314
(703) 739-2782

ASTA WEST COAST OFFICE
4420 Hotel Circle Court, Suite 230
San Diego, CA 92180
(619) 298-5056

AMERICAN RETAIL TRAVEL ASSOCIATION
25 S. Riverside Avenue
Croton on Hudson, NY 10520
(914) 271-HELP

Remember to ask if there are any additional charges for arranging a trip. Some agencies bill clients for long distance phone calls, cables, or other services. Also, always ask about any restrictions or cancellation fees which may apply to your tickets or reservations. Finally, be sure to let your agent know from the beginning that you are a mature adult and, as such, are entitled to all senior discounts available.

DOING IT YOURSELF

If you decide to plan your own trip always ask for the "senior citizen discount" when making your reservations, at the time of purchase or before you check-in. If you wait until you pick up your tickets or check out, it might be too late. Some hotels do not give a senior citizen discount if reservations are booked through a travel agent because they are paying two discounts, a 10 percent travel agent's commission and a 10 percent (or more) senior citizen discount. Also, be aware that you can save money by using toll-free numbers to reserve hotel rooms in hundreds of destinations. The (800) directory assistance operator (800-555-1212) will give you the toll-free numbers.

Some discounts may apply only between certain hours, on certain days of the week, or during specific seasons of the year. Check this out before making reservations.

Don't always take the over-50 discount without inquiring about other available rates. Sometimes special promotional discounts, available to anybody at any age, turn out to have better savings. Ask the reservationist or ticket seller to find you the lowest possible rate at that time.

Since many mature adults look younger than their chronological age, it is particularly important to carry identification with your proof of age (driver's license, passport, resident alien card, Medicare card, senior I.D. card, birth certificate) or membership in an over-50 organization such as AARP or Mature Outlook.

Traveling can be among the most rewarding experiences of your life if you plan ahead and "learn the ropes"!

TRAVEL AGENCIES, CLUBS, AND ORGANIZATIONS FOR 50+ TRAVELERS

Some travel agencies and organizations cater solely to mature travelers. They offer trips and vacations for the fiercely independent or those who enjoy the companionship of tour groups. There are so many choices for the mature traveler today that the only problem is making a decision on where to go.

Here are some companies whose expertise in senior travel has helped thousands of older adults enjoy memorable, well planned trips:

GRAND CIRCLE TRAVEL— 347 Congress Street, Boston, Massachusetts 02210, (617) 350-7500, (800) 221-2610. This company is a direct marketer of international travel for mature adults over 50. They offer escorted tours and cruises, including an Around the World Tour, Live Abroad Vacations, Grand Circle programs, and Countryside Tours. They also offer a free travel-tips brochure called "Going Abroad: 101 Tips for the Mature Traveler," as well as grand tour catalogs and free travel counseling.

GOLDEN AGE TRAVELERS —Pier 27, The Embarcadero, San Francisco, CA 94111, (800) 652-1683. This over-50 travel agency/club focuses mostly on booking cruise trips all over the world. The cost of joining is $10 a year, $15 per couple. Members receive a monthly newsletter listing travel discounts on cruises, trips and land tours.

SAGA INTERNATIONAL HOLIDAYS, LTD.—120 Boylston Street, Boston, MA 02116, (800) 336-SAGA. SAGA (sometimes referred to as "Send a Granny Away") is a well-established travel agency in Great Britain. They specialize in making travel plans for people over 60. Trips can be booked through direct mail or telephone only, since there are no travel agents representing them in this country. SAGA has become very popular with American travelers because of the opportunities they offer for traveling with mature adults from other countries such as Great Britain and Australia. A three-year membership costs $5. Members receive travel discounts, a bi-monthly magazine called *Connections*, opportunities for social gatherings, and a list of "Penfriends" and "Partnership" to help find travel companions and meet people through the mail.

AJS TRAVEL CONSULTANTS, INC.—177 Beach & 116th Street, Rockaway Park, NY 11694, (800) 945-5900. Offers "The 50 Plus Club" which specializes in leisurely paced, escorted tour packages to places such as Switzerland, Italy, and Israel. Tours are discounted.

MAYFLOWER TOURS—1225 Warren Avenue, P.O. Box 490, Downers Grove, IL 60515, (708) 960-3430, (800) 323-7604. Mayflower targets mature travelers 55 or over by offering leisurely paced, fully escorted trips including tours to Hawaii, the Canadian Rockies, and Georgia's Golden Isles. Special trips allow grandparents and grandchildren to travel together. Participants travel by air conditioned motorcoach, stay in quality hotels, and eat meals with others in the tour. If you are a single traveler, Mayflower will find you a roommate as long as you make your reservations 30 days in advance.

MATURE OUTLOOK TRAVEL ALERT—Mature Outlook, 6001 N. Clark Street, Chicago, IL 60660, (800) 336-6330. This over-50 club run by Sears, offers the Travel Alert program, which allows members to sign up for unsold spaces or last-minute cancellations on scheduled trips and tours. These last-minute holidays offer considerable discounts, but you must be ready to leave with very little notice. Membership includes subscriptions in *Mature Outlook* magazine and *The Mature Outlook Newsletter*.

AARP TRAVEL SERVICE—5855 Green Valley Circle, Culver City, CA 90230, (800) 227-7737. AARP members have a variety of travel benefits from which to choose, including escorted tours, trips and cruises to locations all over the globe at discounted group rates. Memberships in AARP cost $5/year and includes the bi-monthly publication Modern Maturity and the *AARP News Bulletin*. Minimum age is 50.

If you belong to an organization like AARP or Mature Outlook, some of these bargains are yours at age 50. Others come along a little later at varying birthdays, so watch for the cutoff points. In many cases, if the person purchasing the ticket qualifies for the minimum age requirement, others sharing the same accommodations are entitled to the same reduced rates.

WHERE TO STAY: HOTEL, MOTEL, AND RESORT BARGAINS

Today's mature traveler has more choices of accommodations than ever before. Almost anywhere you go you will find a senior discount. Whether your make reservations yourself or through a travel agent, consider the following:

- Hotels, motels, and resorts often offer even better discounts if you belong to a recognized senior organization or discount airline program. Remember to ask at what age the senior discount begins.

- When calling for reservations know the dates, arrival time, number of people in your party, price range, type and quality of room you prefer (including amenities and extras: nonsmoking rooms, free complimentary breakfasts, health and fitness centers, indoor pools and jacuzzis, facilities for the handicapped.)

- Whenever possible use (800) toll-free numbers to book reservations through a central operator.

- Always ask about the senior citizen discount at the time you make reservations and when you check-in. Hotel/motels discounts range from 10 percent to as high as 50 percent off regular room rates.

- Request a written confirmation or a reservation confirmation number and bring it when you check in. Also consider guaranteeing your reservation by prepaying the first night (either by credit card or check). By doing this, whether you use it or not, you are guaranteed a reservation that will be held for you even if you arrive late.

- Another way to guarantee your reservation is to prepay through a travel voucher from your travel agent. Visa, MasterCard, and other major credit card companies now issue these through travel agents. To use a travel voucher, simply present it when you check in.

Accommodations for today's mature traveler run the range of price and comfort levels. Prices range from $5 up to several hundred dollars a night depending on your preferences. Listed below are examples of national and international lodging organizations offering senior discounts:

BEST WESTERN. Best Western has more than 3,300 independently owned hotels, inns and resorts across the United States and abroad. Most of the affiliates offer a 10 percent senior discount if you are 55 or over. AARP members receive a 10 percent discount on room rates. Advance reservations are recommended. Call (800) 528-1234.

BUDGET HOST INNS. Located across the United States and Canada, this chain of inns offers senior citizen discounts that vary from inn to inn. Write for a free Budget Host Inn Travel Directory, which includes senior citizen bonus coupons, toll-free Budget Host reservation numbers and a listing of all inns: Budget Host Inns, 2601 Jacksboro Highway, Caravan Suite 202, P.O. Box 10656, Fort Worth, Texas 76114 or call (800) 283-4678 or (800) 835-7427.

BUDGETEL INNS. This inexpensive motel chain offers a 10 percent discount in many of its establishments, if you are over 55. Budgetel Inns are located across the South and Midwest in about 20 states. Confirm your discount when making reservations. Call (800) 428-3438.

CANADIAN PACIFIC HOTELS. Offers special senior citizen discounts at participating hotels. They also offer special weekend rates. Call (800) 828-7447.

COLONY HOTELS AND RESORTS. Offers a 20 percent discount if you are over 59 and a 25 percent discount if you are a member of AARP. Includes 35 hotel, resort, time-share, and condominium properties located in seven states and on five Hawaiian Islands. Call (800) 367-6046.

COMPRI HOTELS. Along with a 15 percent discount, if you are 60 or an AARP member, breakfast is included. There over 20 hotels located in major cities in the United States and Canada. Call (800)426-6774.

COUNTRY HEARTH INNS. A chain of inexpensive motels that offer a 10 percent discount if you are over 50. Call (800) 848-5767.

DAYS INNS. This large chain has over 1,000 properties in the United States, Canada, Mexico, the Netherlands, and France. Days Inns has a special "September Days Club" for people over 50. Membership is $12 a year per person or couple. Members receive 15 to 50 percent off rooms at participating establishments and 10 percent off purchases at gift shops and meals at Days Inns restaurants. September Days members are entitled to group rates on trips and escorted tours, discounts on rental cars, discounted prescription drugs, vehicle insurance plan, discounts at theme parks, free luggage tags, information on last-minute travel opportunities and a free subscription to *Golden Years* magazine. Call (800) 241-5050.

DOUBLETREE HOTELS. Offers the "Silver Leaf" program to travelers 50 and over for a 15 percent discount on lodging. Call (800)528-0444.

DRURY INNS. If you are over 55 or a member of AARP, Drury Inns offer 10 percent discounts on regular rooms at all locations. Call (800) 325-8300.

ECONOMY INNS OF AMERICA. This chain is located in California, Georgia, and Florida and offers 10 percent discount to guests over 55 or to AARP members. Call (800) 826-0778.

EMBASSY SUITES HOTELS. If you are over 65, a member of AARP, National Retired Teachers Association, National Council of Senior Citizens, or have a Silver Savers Passport, you receive a 10 percent discount on their two-room suites. Complimentary breakfast and cocktails are also included. Call (800) 362-2779.

25

EXEL INNS OF AMERICA, INC. Located in Illinois, Texas, Wisconsin, Minnesota, and Iowa, these inns offer a 10 percent senior citizen discount on room rates, if you are 55 or over. Call (800) 356-8013.

HAMPTON INNS. Offers a special membership program for people over 50. The "Lifestyle 50" program entitles guests to share a room with three other travelers 50+ for the one-person rate. The "Lifestyle 50" program is honored at any of the 220 Hampton Inns across the United states. Call (800) HAMPTON.

HARLEY HOTELS. 10 percent discount at all of these luxury hotels for members of AARP. Call (800) 321-2323.

HILTON HOTELS. Offers the Hilton "Senior HHonors Program." Members are entitled to up to 50 percent off room rates, plus meal discounts (even if you're not a hotel guest) at 240 Hilton restaurants and credit certificates for participating hotels. Membership is $45/year or $75 for life. Call (800) 842-4242 or write to Senior HHonors Service Center, 2050 Chennault Drive, Carrollton, TX 75006.

HOLIDAY INNS AND HOLIDAY INN CROWNE PLAZA HOTELS. Guests 55 and over or members of AARP, receive a 10 percent discount on all room rates at over 1,000 participating hotels. Members of Sears' Mature Outlook receive 20 percent off room rates and 10 percent off meal bills at any Holiday Inn restaurants. Call (800) HOLIDAY.

HOWARD JOHNSON. If you are 60 or over or a member of a national senior organization, Howard Johnson offers "Howard Johnson Road Rally." Members are entitled to up to 50 percent off regular rooms. Non-members can call ahead for reservations and receive 15 percent off room rates. Call (800) 634-3464.

HYATT HOTELS. Each of these independently owned hotel offers its own senior discounts. Discounts ranging from 10 to 50 percent off room rates for up to four persons sharing a room. Call (800) 233-1234.

IMPERIAL 400 INNS. Offers 10 percent off to those 55 and over and members of national senior citizen organizations. Call (800) 368-4400.

INN SUITES. This chain, located in the West, has a special program for senior citizens 55 and over called "The Silver Passport Program." Members receive 10 to 15 percent off regular room rates. Call (800) 842-4242.

KARENA HOTELS, INC. These hotels include certain Ramada, Econolodge, and Rodeway Inns located mainly in Florida. Members enrolled in their "Silver Club" (for age 50 and over) receive a 20 percent discount off regular room rates, free luggage tags, and a free coupon book with travel discounts. Call (800) 365-6935.

KNIGHTS INN. With 110 locations in the Southeast, this motel chain gives a 10 percent discount to anyone 55 and over. Call (614) 755-6230.

LA QUINTA MOTOR INNS. Receive a 20 percent discount on room rates if you are 60 and over or a member of AARP (plus a $10 membership fee). 200 locations across the Sunbelt. Call (800) 531-5900.

L-K MOTELS. Offers a 10 percent discount for anybody 55 and over or for members of AARP. Call (800) 848-5767.

MARRIOTT. Marriott's Leisure Life Program. If you are 62, or 50 and a member of AARP, you get 50 percent off weekday regular rates at over 100 locations in the United States, Canada, and cities abroad and you also get a 25 percent discount on dining and 10 percent discount on gift-shop purchases. Call (800) 228-9290.

NENDELS MOTOR INNS. Receive 10 percent off regular room rates if you are 60 or over or a member of a national senior organization. Locations in the Pacific Northwest. Call (800) 547-0106.

OMNI HOTELS. Thirty-eight locations in the United States offer 50 percent discount on regular room rates to AARP members. Advance reservations suggested. Call (800) 843-6664.

THE POINTE—MOUNTAINSIDE RESORTS. These three resorts in Phoenix offer a "Prime Time" senior citizen discount program to guests 50 or over. Members are entitled to up to 50 percent off $120 to $135 suites. Includes breakfast and free cocktail reception. Call (800) 8-POINTE.

QUALITY INNS/COMFORT INNS/CLARION INNS/RODEWAY INNS/ECONO LODGES/FRIENDSHIP INNS/SLEEP INNS (Choice Hotels Int'l). With over 3,000 hotels worldwide, Choice Hotels International offers a year round "Prime Time" program. If you are 60+ or a member of AARP, you are eligible for the Super Saver rate of 10 to 30 percent off the room rate. Call (800) 221-2222.

RADISSON HOTELS. If you are 65 or over or are a member of a senior organization you and your roommates receive a 25 percent discount on regular room rates. Advance reservations necessary. Call (800) 228-9822.

RAMADA INN. Ramada offers its "Best Years Program" if you are over 59 or are a member of a senior organization. Members are entitled to a 15 to 25 percent discount on room rates at nearly 500 participating establishments. Call (800) 272-6232.

RED CARPET INNS/MASTER HOSTS INNS/SCOTTISH INNS. Offers a year round 10 percent discount on room rates to guests 55 and over or members of AARP or NRT. Call (800) 251-1062.

RED LION INNS/THUNDERBIRD MOTOR INNS. Guests 50 and over who present a senior organization card or an AARP card, receive 20 percent off regular room rates. Advanced reservations suggested. Call (800) 547-8010.

RED ROOF INNS. Offers a new senior savings program "Redi Card +60" which entitles members to a 10 percent discount on room rates, plus discounts on future stays at Red Roof Inns, a quarterly newsletter, and Rand McNally road map. Call (800) 843-7663.

SHERATON HOTELS. Located in over 62 countries, participating Sheraton Hotels offer a 25 percent discount on most room rates to those over 60 or AARP members. Ask for the discount when making reservations. Call (800) 325-3535.

SONESTA INTERNATIONAL HOTELS. If you are a member of AARP, you will receive a 10 to 15 percent discount off room rates at any of their 13 deluxe hotels. Make sure to request your discount when making reservations. Call (800) 343-7170.

STOUFFER HOTELS. This hotel chain offers a "Great Years Program" that gives senior citizens 59 and over up to 50 percent discount off regular room rates. Available only at participating Stouffer Hotels. Call (800) HOTELS-1.

SUPER 8 MOTELS, INC. Over 700 Super 8 Motels across the United States and Canada offer a 10 percent discount for senior travelers 55 or over. Call (800) 843-1991.

TRAVELODGE AND DISCOUNT HOTELS. Participating locations offer a 15 percent discount on room rates to members of most senior organizations. "The Classic Travel Club" ($15 a year, $25 for two years, $35 for three years) entitles members to receive 20 percent off regular room rates. Call (800) 255-3050 or write to Classic Travel Club, P.O. Box 93020, Long Beach, CA 90809-3020.

TREADWAY INNS. Save from 10 to 15 percent off room rates from this small Eastern hotel chain if you are a member of a senior organization or 55 and over. Call (800) 631-0182.

VAGABOND INNS. Guests 55 and over who join the "Vagabond Inns' Club 55", receive 10 to 15 percent off regular room rates plus other benefits. Membership fee is $10. Call (800) 522-1555 or write: The Vagabond Inns Club, P.O. Box 85011, San Diego, CA 92138.

WESTIN HOTELS AND RESORTS. This luxury hotel chain offers discounts up to 50 percent off regular room rates. Advance reservations are required. Each hotel has its own discount policy. Members of United Airlines' Silver Wings get a 50 percent discount, based on availability.

The Peabody Hotel in Orlando, Florida offers an innovative senior discount program: dollars for years credit against regular guest room prices for anyone 50 and over. For example, if you are 50, you receive $50 off; if you are 60, you get $60 off, and if you are 100, you receive $100. In addition, children and grandchildren up to 18 can share your room for free, or you can book them a separate room at a 50 percent discount. Call (800) PEABODY for details.

Always check for a senior citizen discount, even if you are booking into an independently owned establishment. You have nothing to lose by asking, and you may find they offer considerable savings in order to stay competitive with the chain operators.

IF YOU DON'T WANT TO STAY IN A HOTEL

If you are innovative, imaginative and will consider alternative sources of lodging, the following possibilities can also save you money in your travels.

INNter Lodging

INNter Lodging is a co-op organization. Members stay in a choice of homes across the United States and Canada at very little cost. Members must agree to make their homes available to other travelers at least four months of the year. For information write to INNter Lodging Co-op, Tacoma, Washington 98407; or call (206)756-0343.

Servas

Servas is an international cooperative system of hosts and travelers established to help build world peace, good will, and understanding. It provides a list of hosts (all over the United Sates and the rest of the world), along with their activities and interests. Simply share your home with others in return for their hospitality when you travel to their home. Write to Servas, 11 John Street, New York, NY 10038, or call (212) 267-0252.

YMCA's

The YMCA offers inexpensive accommodations throughout North America that are safe, comfortable, and conveniently located. You should make reservations several months in advance due to their popularity. Included is your room, use of swimming pool, exercise facilities, and library. Some Y's offer package programs that include breakfast, some other meals, and sightseeing. Write: The Y's Way, 356 West 34th Street, New York, NY 10001.

Auto-Truck Stops

Full-service truck stops offer inexpensive, comfortable hotel rooms. Some include amenities such as laundromats, restaurants, barber-shops, and convenience stores. First priority for available rooms is reserved for truckers.

Campus Accommodations

Colleges and universities across the United States, Canada, and Europe rent rooms to travelers in the summertime and during school vacations. The cost is minimal, and some include breakfast and use of campus facilities. Contact the housing office of colleges in areas you plan to visit or get a copy of "U.S. and Worldwide Accommodations Guide" ($11.95). Write to Campus Travel Service, P.O. Box 5007, Laguna Beach, CA 92652 or call (714) 497-3044.

Oakwood Resort Apartments

These resort apartments may be rented by mature travelers 55 and over. They are located in metropolitan areas in California, Nevada, Washington D.C., Georgia, Virginia, North Carolina, Texas, and Colorado. They must be rented for 30 days or more, and if rented between November and February, there is a substantial discount. The apartments are completely furnished, including kitchen utensils, and linens. Most locations have tennis courts, fitness centers, swimming pools, and club houses. Write to: R&B Enterprises, 2222 Corinth Ave., Los Angeles, CA 90064, or call (800) 421-6654.

Camping

According to a recent survey by the camping industry, the number of campers who are retirees is increasing. And as they continue to grow, will be requiring more conveniences and a greater choice of recreational activities. There are public campgrounds, private campgrounds, primitive, and luxurious resort campgrounds. Many are located near historic points of interest, major attractions or within state and national parks. Prices range from as low as $1.50 to $20 per night. Amenities include fireplaces, picnic tables, flush toilets, showers, electricity, running water, grocery stores, dumping stations, and coin laundries.

To receive a *National Parks: Camping Guide* write to: Superintendent of Documents, U.S. Government Printing Office, Dept. 33, Washington, D.C. 20402. Enclose $3.50. For other camping information write: National Park Service, Office of Public Inquiries, P.O. Box 37127, Washington, D.C. 20013-7127.

For information about Kampgrounds Of America (KOA), the largest chain of privately owned campgrounds in the U.S. send for the *KOA Handbook and Directory*. Write: Kampgrounds of America, 550 N. 31st Street, 4th Floor, Billings, Montana 59101, or call (406) 248-7444, or pick up a directory at your nearest KOA campground.

Another multi-site campground operation, YOGI BEAR'S JELLYSTONE PARK CAMP RESORTS AND SAFARI CAMP-GROUND has a free directory. To receive a copy write: Leisure Systems, Inc, Route 209, Bushkill, PA 18324.

For more information about camping in the U.S. write for: *Trailer Life RV Campground and Services Directory*, 29901 Agoura Road, Agoura, CA 91301 or *Wheelers RV Resort and Campground Guide*, 1310 Jarvis, Elk Grove, Illinois 60007.

A highly successful international organization, THE GOOD SAM CLUB, offers discounts and benefits to owners of recreational vehicles. Although membership is open to all ages, the majority of those belonging are over 50. Over 2,000 local chapters host outings, hold meetings and schedule regular campouts. Savings and services include:

> 10 percent discount at 1,600 RV parks and campgrounds; 10 percent discounts on RV parts and accessories; Emergency road service (includes towing); RV vehicle insurance; Health insurance; Subscriptions to *Trailer Life* and *MotorHome* magazines; Trip routing service; Mail forwarding service; Credit card protection; Lost pet service and lost key service.

With all these benefits and a membership fee of $19 a year, The Good Sam Club is a bargain for folks who spend a lot of time on the road. They also organize "caraventure" tours all over the world. For information: The Good Sam Club, P.O. Box 500, Agoura, CA 91301; (800) 423-5061; (in CA) (800) 382-3455.

Bed and Breakfasts

There are so many wonderful bed & breakfast accommodations located in the United States and abroad that it would be impossible to try and list them. For the most current information regarding bed and breakfast establishments in areas you plan to visit, contact the tourist agencies in those areas or check your local bookstore or library for bed and breakfast directories.

EVERGREEN BED & BREAKFAST CLUB, 1926 South Pacific Coast Highway, Redondo Beach, California 90277, (301) 261-0180. The Evergreen Bed & Breakfast Club is designed for those mature travelers over 50 willing to give up rooms in their homes to other travelers. Club members provide guest rooms for fellow members traveling throughout the United States, Canada, and Europe. There are presently over 600 homes in the Evergreen Club. Membership cost $50 per couple or $40 for singles. Members receive annual directories and a quarterly news-letter. The directory gives names, addresses, occupations, interests, policies on smoking and pets and a listing of special attractions in the area. Rates are generally $10-single or $15-double per night.

More Clubs For Mature Travelers

GOLDEN COMPANIONS, P.O. Box 754, Pullman, Washington 99163-0754. This organization is for those senior travelers who prefer to travel with a companion or in a small group. Golden Companions operates a travel companion network and publishes a newsletter exclusively for those travelers over 50 years old. Membership includes a bimonthly newsletter *The Golden Traveler*, the networking service, a complete membership list (nearly 1,000) a confidential mail exchange, tour dis-counts, and vacation-home exchanges.

PARTNERS-IN-TRAVEL, P.O. Box 491145, Los Angeles, CA 90049, (213) 476-4869. Partners-in-Travel, open to all ages, offers single travelers an opportunity to connect with other travelers for friendship and savings on the cost of travel. A $40 annual membership package includes a bimonthly newsletter with free listings for members seeking travel companions, free counseling, free listings of home-exchange, and a special publication, *To Your Good Health*.

TRAVEL COMPANIONS EXCHANGE, P.O. Box 833-M, Amityville, NY 11701, (516) 454-0880, will also match up single travelers for a small fee. Other organizations offering similar services include: *Travel Mates*, New York, NY; *Singleworld*, New York, NY; *Travel Partners Club*, Crystal River, FL; and *Travel Buddy*, Minneapolis, MN.

LONERS ON WHEELS, P.O. Box 1355, Poplar Bluff, Missouri, 63901. This 54-chapter national recreation club is a social club for RV owners who are single. The club targets mainly seniors and retirees. Remaining single is the rule of the road or you are automatically dropped. Numerous campouts, recreational and educational activities, and rallies are announced in a monthly newsletter.

LONERS OF AMERICA, 191 Villa Del Rio Blvd., Boca Raton, FL 33432. This is another club for single RVers. There are more than 1,200 members throughout the country, ranging in age from their 40s to 90s. They hold campouts, meetings, rallies, and caravans all over the country. Members receive an annual membership directory and newsletter detailing events and activities.

AMERICAN JEWISH CONGRESS, 15 E. 84th Street, New York, NY 10028, (800) 221-4694, (212) 879-4588. This organization offers tours to Israel for single travelers who join other similarly aged solo travelers. Every year they offer two departures for singles between ages of 39 and 55, and four trips for solo travelers over the age of 55.

FLY AND SAVE MONEY

Most airlines offer senior citizens discounts of at least 10 percent off regular fares (you can fly first class for free if you can prove you are 100 years old!). However, these fares often cost more than if you used excursion fares, also referred to as SuperSaver, MaxSaver, and Ultra-Saver fares, where the discount may be 50 percent or more. Often "limited time only" promotional fares offer even more savings (up to 80 percent) at certain times when airlines are looking to fill seats. There is no difference between the seating, service, or aircraft on a full-coach or economy ticket and a excursion/promotional fare ticket. However, there are usually only a certain number of these cut-price seats available on each flight, so it is important to book as early as possible. In fact, if you are going to use your senior discount with a SuperSaver fare, you will most likely be required to make your reservations at least 30 days in advance.

SuperSaver and MaxSaver fares carry a number of important restrictions. There are usually hefty cancellations fees, blackout periods, a 7 to 30-day advance purchase requirement, a 24-hour payment requirement, round-trip purchase requirement, Saturday night stayover, and other conditions. Always ask about all applicable restrictions before purchasing your tickets. You need to decide whether these limitations and inconveniences are worth the savings. If you are flexible in your plans, they usually are.

There are four ways airlines are currently using to attract mature travelers:

1. Clubs with discounts (frequent flyers).
2. Straight discounts.
3. Unlimited-mileage passes.
4. Coupon books.

The minimum age for discount senior fares is 50, usually honored in conjunction with proof of membership in AARP. However, check with individual airlines since some offer senior rates starting at age 60 or older. Most programs allow a companion of any age, regardless of sex or relationship to travel at the same reduced fare.

When choosing among the confusing, ever-changing fares airlines offer, always ask for the lowest current fare (whether you're using a travel agent or working directly with the airline reservationist). Check local newspaper advertisements, travel magazines, or one of the several excellent travel newsletters for the latest promotional offers.

Let them know that you qualify for a senior discount, but be aware that you may get a better deal by going with a special promotion or supersaver fare. Sometimes your senior discount can cut these low fares even lower. You may even get lucky and hit a special promotional fare for seniors (these are usually run during off-peak seasons). These fares are often significantly lower than other fares and may be the cheapest way to go.

Yearly passes and discount coupon books are available for seniors who do a significant amount of traveling. Before purchasing either of these options, however, it is important to determine how many trips you're likely to be making over the next year. Coupon booklets can be purchased in four or eight-coupon sets, each coupon being good for a one-way domestic flight. Seven to fourteen day advance reservations are nearly always required.

Most coupons are good for all destinations that an airline flies within the continental United States. Travel to Alaska or Hawaii usually requires using two coupons. However, if you don't think you'll be doing enough flying with a single airline to justify the cash outlay, you may be better off with regular senior citizen discounts or searching out MaxSaver fares. The same rule for frequent flying applies to buying a multi-use domestic or international "passport" or air pass from an airline.

Be prepared to present a valid proof of age or club/airline membership card at the check-in counter. If you don't look your age, and don't have proof with you, your discount may not be honored, and you'll end up spending more time and money at the check-in counter.

The following are examples of senior discounts currently offered by airline companies.

AMERICAN AIRLINES —(800) 433-7300. American Airlines/American Eagle offers three senior citizen discount programs:

1. 10 percent Senior TrAAveler Discount if you are 62 or older. Discount is valid at all times and may also be applied to a companion ticket.

2. Senior TrAAvelers coupon books can be purchased by travelers 62 or older. Four one-way 2,000 mile coupons cost $473; eight coupons cost $791.

3. Special Discount for AARP members. Members receive a 10 percent discount off lowest-published round-trip fares, including promotional fares, for flights within the United States, the Caribbean, and Mexico.

CONTINENTAL AIRLINES—(800) 525-0280; (800) 441-1135 Senior fares . If you are 62 or over, you are eligible for a 10 percent discount on all fares on Continental. The "Freedom Passport" discount program allows folks 62 to fly Continental's routes in the United States, Canada, and the U.S. Virgin Islands for one year for a single price of $1,299. A first-class passport costs $1,699. Global passports cost $2,699, and $4,699, respectively, for coach and first class and are valid throughout the continental United States, Mexico, the Caribbean, Central America, Hawaii, Europe, and the Pacific.

Continental also has the "Freedom Trip" program for travelers 62 and over with booklets of four one-way coupons for $449 or eight one-way coupons for $749. Coupons are valid for travel to all destinations in the mainland United States, Alaska, or Hawaii (two coupons required for Alaska and Hawaii).

DELTA AIRLINES—(800) 221-1212. Delta Airlines offers a 10 percent senior citizen discount for seniors 62 or over and a traveling companion of any age on the lowest available fares. Their "Young at Heart" discount plan includes coupon booklets of four for $472 or eight for $790, each coupon being good for one-way reserved seat travel to all U.S. cities including Hawaii, Alaska, and San Juan. Booklets are valid for one year from the date of purchase.

MIDWEST EXPRESS AIRLINES, INC.—(800) 452-2022. For those 65 and over with proof of age, a 10 percent discount is given on all fares to all destinations. Members of the Golden Travel Club receive frequent-flyer benefits as well as the senior discount.

NORTHWEST AIRLINES—800) 225-2525. Offers three discount programs for senior travelers 62 or over:

1. "WorldHorizons" program. 10 percent senior citizen discount off most domestic fares, for travelers 62 or over. No membership fee and all flights earn frequent-flyer credit.

2. "Senior Ultrafare." Travelers 62 or over can purchase four or eight one-way discount coupon booklets for flights in the continental United States and Canada (Alaska or Hawaii flights require two coupons). Guest certificates entitle accompanying companion to reduced fares. Four-coupon book costs $472; eight-coupon book, $790.

3. "WorldPerks Senior." Members get a free trip every 20,000 miles and additional benefits and discounts including newsletter, hotel, car rental, cruise discounts, and reduced fee in WorldClub membership. Contact your travel agent or call Northwest Airlines Reservations at (800) 225-2525 to enroll.

PAN AMERICAN WORLD AIRWAYS—(800) 221-1111; (800) 252-8879 for ValuePass. Travelers 62 or over and a younger companion receive 10 percent off any published fares within the United States and Europe. Pan American also offers four levels of their "ValuePass," giving varying numbers of trips to different destinations for one price. Senior travelers get 10 percent off regular pass price. Trips include travel to the Caribbean, Latin America, Mexico, Europe, and destinations in the United States. Other benefits include discounts on hotels and car rentals. Call for the current price information.

TWA—(800) 221-2000; (800) 872-8374 for Takeoff Pass.

1. Travelers 62 or over receive a 10 percent discount on most flights in the United States, Puerto Rico, and Europe. A traveling companion of any age receives the same discount.

2. For travelers 62 or over, TWA offers the "Senior Travel Pak," their discount coupon program. Four one-way coupons ($396) valid for travel to any TWA destination within the continental United States or between the United States and the Caribbean Two coupons required for Hawaii. The Senior Travel Pak also offers the "Europe Bonus Option Certificate," one round-trip coupon to Europe for $449. Includes a choice of 21 cities in Europe. Call TWA for details and restrictions.

3. Also for travelers 62 or over, TWA offers their "Takeoff Pass" at a 10 percent discount. This entitles you to a year of travel that includes one round-trip vacation to Hawaii, Europe, the Bahamas, or Puerto Rico, and three round trips anywhere in the continental United States. Call to confirm current "Takeoff Pass" prices.

UNITED AIRLINES—(800) 241-6522; (800) 628-2868 for Silver Wings Plus Travel Club.

1. Travelers 62 or over receive 10 percent off coach/economy round-trip fares.

2. Travelers 62 or over can join United's "Silver Wings Plus Travel Club." A $50 membership fee ($100 for the Companion Membership), entitles travelers to a 10 percent discount on United Airlines and United Express fares to the United States, Thailand, Korea, Germany, Canada, Philippines, China, Hong Kong, Australia, Taiwan, New Zealand, Singapore, France, Mexico, and Singapore. Program is also valid on Alitalia, British Airways, Sabena, Iberia, and KLM flights. Members are entitled to 10 to 50 percent discounts on Clarion Hotels, Westin Hotels and Resorts, Hyatt Hotels and Resorts, Comfort Inns, Quality Inns, Renaissance Hotels, and Ramada Inns. Other benefits include discounts on

Hertz, Alamo, and Dollar rental cars, a $25 discount certificate, and a quarterly travel magazine.

3. Senior travel coupons. Four one-way 2,000 mile coupons cost $473; eight one-way coupons cost $790. Valid every day. Two coupons required for Alaska and Hawaii. Good for travel to all U.S. cities, including San Juan.

USAIR—(800) 428-4322.

1. If you are 62 or over, USAir offers the Senior Saver Fare for a 10 percent discount on domestic and Canadian flights and commuter flights. Companions of any age receive same discount.

2. Senior Saver discount books. For travelers 62 or over, four one-way coupons ($473) or eight one-way coupons ($790) valid for travel to any destination within the continental Unites States plus San Juan. Senior Saver discount books are good for one year from the date of purchase.

U.S. Regional Airlines

ALASKA AIRLINES—(800) 426-0333. If you are 62 or over, Alaska Airlines offers a 10 percent senior citizen discount on any published fare. A companion of any age traveling with you receives the same discount. Senior discount coupon books are available for travel within the United States and Canada. Four one-way coupons ($472) or eight one-way coupons ($790). Travel to Alaska requires using two coupons each direction.

ALOHA AIRLINES—(800) 367-5250. Flies within the Hawaiian Islands. Aloha Airlines offer 10 percent off one-way fares for those over 60.

AMERICA WEST—(800) 833-8602 (senior fares); Senior fares gives travelers 62 or over discounts between 10 and 50 percent off normal coach fares depending on route taken. American West also offers the "Senior Saver Packs," discount booklets of four one-way coupons ($430) or eight one-way coupons ($720). Coupons are valid to all U.S. cities including Hawaii. Two coupons are needed for Hawaii and travel to or from East Coast cities. Coupon booklets are good for one year.

HAWAIIAN AIR—(800) 367-5320. This interisland airline offers senior discounts between 7 and 9 percent if you are 60 or over.

MIDWAY AIRLINES—(800) 621-5700. Travelers 62 or over receive special senior discounts on flights between 9 A.M. and 3 P.M., Monday through Thursday and all day Saturday. There is also a coupon program good for flights to all Southwest destinations. Fares range from $19 to $79 one-way. Coupons are valid every day with no advance purchase required.

Canadian Airlines

The following airlines in Canada offer 10 to 50 percent discounts for senior citizens 62 and over with proof of age. Companions traveling on the same itinerary also receive the discount. Ask whether discounts apply during the time you plan to travel.

AIR CANADA—(800) 776-3000.
CANADIAN AIRLINES INTERNATIONAL—(800) 426-7000.

Foreign Airlines

ALITALIA—(800) 223-5730. If you are 65 or over and a member of United Airlines "Silver Wings Plus Travel Club," Alitalia offers you a 10 percent discount on any flight.

BRITISH AIRWAYS—(800) 247-9297. Offers the Privileged Traveller Program (60 or over), which entitles members to a 10 percent senior discount on all air fares. There are no penalties for cancellations or changed itineraries (before the day prior to departure) and no blackout periods. Members also receive a 10 percent discount on all Venice-Simplon Orient Express departures, and British Airway Holiday Tours.

EL AL—(800) 223-6700 or (212) 768-9200 in NY If you are 60 or over, you are eligible for a 15 percent discount on El Al flights.

FINNAIR—(800) 777-5553. If you are 65 or over, Finnair offers special senior discounts on flights from Los Angeles or New York to Helsinki. Check Finnair for costs and limitations.

IBERIA—(800) 772-4642. If you are 65 or over and a member of United Airlines "Silver Wings Plus Travel Club," Iberia Airlines offers you a 10 percent discount off their fares.

KLM ROYAL DUTCH AIRLINES—(800) 777-5553. If you are 65 or over and a member of United Airlines "Silver Wings Plus Travel Club," KLM Airlines offers you a 10 percent discount on any flight. Also KLM lowers the fares in the off-season for those 65 or over on flights to many cities in the Netherlands.

LUFTHANSA—(800) 645-3880. If you are 62 or over, Lufthansa offers 10 percent discounts on their fares.

MEXICANA—(800) 531-7921. If you are 62 or over, Mexicana offers 10 percent senior discounts on one-way or round-trip fares from the United States to Mexico and domestic travel within Mexico. One traveling companion of any age receive same rate. Check for holiday blackout periods.

TAP AIR PORTUGAL—(800) 221-7370. Offers small senior discounts for those over 60 (and their companions) traveling during off-peak times.

SCANDINAVIAN AIRLINES (SAS)—(800) 221-2350. Travelers 65 or over receive a discount on some flights within Sweden.

Most major airline travel clubs (including American, Continental, Northwest, TWA, United and USAir) offer special savings for mature adults. There is an initiation fee for membership ranging between $50 and $150. The average fare for a flight ranges from $500 to $700 for members.

TAKE A CRUISE FOR LESS

How do you like the idea of a traveling resort? You unpack once and the rest of your transportation plans are taken care of. A recent survey of American travelers found that almost half of all cruise passengers are over 50. Cruise travel opportunities are nearly endless: Caribbean, Mediterranean, Alaska, South Pacific, the Orient, Hawaii, the Mexican Riviera, Baja California, South America, New England, Eastern Canada, Scandinavia, British Isles, the Mississippi and other rivers, through England, the wine country of France, and the Rivers of Germany. You can cruise just about anywhere there's enough water for a ship.

 Cruises offer some of the best travel bargains available. If you book your cruise far in advance (a year or more) or very close to the date of sailing, you can save a bundle, 50 percent or more off the list price. You can also put yourself on "standby" for an upcoming cruise. Check the travel section of your newspaper for advertisements for last-minute cruise travel.

There are agencies that specialize in last-minute travel that offer deep discounts. Although they are called "last-minute," several of them will book passengers in advance knowing these huge ships usually have space available. A few last-minute travel clubs/agencies that specialize in this type of travel are:

ENCORE SHORT NOTICE, (800) 638-8976

MOMENT'S NOTICE, (213) 486-0505

VACATIONS TO GO, (800) 624-7338

LAST MINUTE TRAVEL CLUB, (617) 267-9800

You can also save if you book through a cruise discounter. In this case, you should be knowledgeable about individual cruise ships, itineraries, cabin locations, etc. A listing of cruise specials called "World of Cruising" is offered free by CRUISE LINE INC., a Miami based discount cruise and information center. For information call (800) 777-0707.

When planning your cruise, ask for special cruise values during "shoulder" (between high and low season) and "off" seasons. The cruise is the same, but the price is less if you can travel during times when the demand is lower.

Cruise costs vary according to destination. For example, the average daily cost per person is $139 along the Mexican Riviera; $149 in the Caribbean; $160 to Bermuda; $180 to Canada/New England; $184 in Europe; $198 to Alaska; and $266 to the Orient. Prices for a cruise include nearly everything: stateroom, lavish meals, entertainment, pool facilities, gymnasium, social programs, some shore tours and other activities. Compare the above prices to the prices you are quoted by you travel agent. As part of their service your travel agent can reserve dinner seating, arrange connecting air and ground transportation, suggest and book pre- and post-cruise tours, and advise on passport and visa requirements.

One of the most interesting concepts in cruises is the "educational" or "special interest" cruise. These cruises offer high-I.Q. itineraries for people who like the convenience of cruising, but want a vacation with more mental stimulation than shipboard bingo, shopping, and shore excursions. These innovative travel programs are offered by cruise lines, museums, university alumni associations and other groups. They feature lecturers, expedition leaders and naturalists who are experts in their fields of interest. Some programs are on expedition ships especially designed to reach remote destinations.

Below are some nonprofit groups and cruise companies that sponsor these types of cruises:

AMERICAN MUSEUM OF NATURAL HISTORY (800) 462-8687

FRIENDS OF THE MUSEUM OF COMPARATIVE ZOOLOGY, HARVARD UNIVERSITY (617) 495-2463

NATIONAL AUDOBON SOCIETY (212) 546-9140

SMITHSONIAN NATIONAL ASSOCIATE PROGRAM (202) 357-4700

STANFORD ALUMNI ASSOCIATION (415) 725-1093

WORLD WILDLIFE FUND EXPEDITIONS (202) 778-9683

CLASSICAL CRUISES (800) 252-7745

CLIPPER CRUISES (800) 325-0010

GALAPAGOS CRUISES (800) 527-2500

RENAISSANCE CRUISES (800) 525-5350

SALEN LINDBLAD CRUISING (800) 223-5688

SOCIETY EXPEDITIONS (800) 426-7794

SPECIAL EXPEDITIONS (800) 762-0003

SWAN HELLENIC CRUISES (800) 426-5492

WORLD EXPLORER CRUISES (800) 854-3935

Most groups say their typical passengers are seasoned travelers around age 55. Although these types of trips are generally not a bargain, they do offer a stimulating, intellectual atmosphere not usually found aboard typical cruise ships.

The following are cruise companies who have trips designed especially for seniors:

CHANDRIS FANTASY CRUISES—(212) 750-0044, (800) 621-3446. Chandris Fantasy Cruises has a "Senior Saver" program for travelers 65 or over, which includes a 50 percent senior citizen discount to the second occupant in a cabin with a passenger who has paid a full fare. The company offers voyages both in the Caribbean and year-round in Europe.

SENIOR-WORLD (Gramercy Travel) —(800) 223-6490. Since Senior-World schedules its voyages during the off seasons (fall and early winter), it can offer great deals with rates well below regular prices. If you are 45 or over, you can travel to Caribbean ports, Cancun or Cozumel in Mexico, and receive first class treatment.

PREMIER CRUISE LINES—(800) 888-6759; in Florida: (407) 783-5061. This is Walt Disney World's official cruise line. The company offers a 10 percent discount to travelers 59 or over. Cruise packages generally include round trip air fare, a three or four night cruise to the Bahamas out of Port Canaveral, Florida, a three or four night stay in a hotel near Disney World, (anybody else who shares your cabin gets the 10 percent discount), plus free admission to Disney's Magic Kingdom, Spaceport USA, Epcot Center, Disney-MGM Studios Theme Park and a rental car with unlimited mileage. A recent promotional offering cost $795 (excluding senior discount) for the entire package, including air fare from the West Coast.

SEA ESCAPE CRUISE LINES—(800) 327-7400; in Florida: (800) 432-0900. This cruise line offers one-day cruises with special discounts for mature travelers over 55 years. Cruise ships leave from Port Canaveral, Fort Lauderdale, St. Petersburg, Miami, and Tampa. The best discounts are in the early summer months between April and June.

SOUTH FLORIDA CRUISES, INC.—(800) 327-SHIP; in Florida: (305) 739-7447. This cruise line specializes in trips to the Far East, Alaska, Europe, Caribbean, Mexico, South Pacific, Panama Canal, and South America with special reduced rates. Senior travelers receive additional savings.

BUS AND RAILROAD EXCURSIONS

Senior citizens 65 and over and handicapped mature travelers are entitled to a 25 percent discount on AMTRAK by presenting appropriate identification. The discounts are not restricted on holidays. There are no requirements to buy closed-end round-trip tickets. The senior discounts apply to any regular one-way fare of $50 or more, but buying a round-trip ticket is the most economical way to go. There is no charge for stopovers on one-way tickets, but you must report a stopover when making ticket reservations.

AMTRAK operates trains and Metroliners that have reserved seating. Coach and club car (first class) seats are available on Metroliners, which service most major Atlantic Coast cities and major metropolitan destinations throughout the United States. Sleeping cars are available between long distances. Snack bars are provided on most trains, and for overnight travel, there are dining cars serving meals during the day and evening. For information contact: Office of Customer Relations, AMTRAK, P.O. Box 2709, Washington, D.C. 20013, or call (800) 872-7245.

If you wish to travel in Canada by train, contact VIA RAIL, Customer Service, 20 King Street West, Floor 5, Toronto, Ontario M5H 1C4, Canada; Tel: (514) 871-6349. They offer a number of all-inclusive tours. Anyone 60 and over receives a 10 percent discount off regular transportation charges. They also offer additional discounts of 40 percent during "off peak" periods.

GREYHOUND/TRAILWAYS offers two senior citizen discount programs: a 10 percent discount to senior citizens 65 and over for trips that begin on Monday, Tuesday, Wednesday, and Thursday, and a 5 percent discount for trips that begin on Friday, Saturday, and Sunday. When making reservations, check for availability of these discounts. Contact: Greyhound/Trailways, 111 West Clarendon Avenue, Phoenix, Arizona 85077-6999, or call your local operator for the nearest Greyhound/Trailways reservation office.

GRAY LINE TOURS motorcoach company operates in cities throughout the United States. It offers 15 percent off half-day and full-day sight-seeing tours to members of AARP and other senior organizations. Call the Gray Line Tours office in your area.

For a list of National Tour Association member companies or information about specific motorcoach tours contact: National Tour Association, Inc., North American Headquarters, P.O. Box 3071, Lexington, KY 40596-3071, or call (800) NTA-8886.

Travelers interested in motorcoach tours can also check with their local Automobile Club Association office for information.

RENTING A CAR

The key to obtaining the best rate when renting a car is to reserve one in advance. When you call about rates or reservations, always have available a valid driver's license, a major credit card, your senior organization's ID number and your own membership card for reference. Never rent a car without getting a discount or a special promotional rate. Always ask for the lowest rate available at that time.

Most major car rental companies have toll-free reservation offices for reserving a car most anywhere in the world. Below are car rental organizations that offer special senior rates or discounts.

ALAMO—(800) 327-9633. Alamo gives discounts on car rentals to senior drivers and members of Classic Travel Club run by Travellodge, Days Inns' September Days Club, AARP, and United Silver Wings. Ask about the "Golden Wheels" program.

AVIS—(800) 331-1800. Avis offers special car rental discounts of 5 to 10 percent to senior citizens and members of Mature Outlook, AARP, and CARP.

BUDGET/SEARS RENT-A-CAR—(800) 527-0700. Offers daily rental discounts of around $5 to members of AARP, Mature Outlook, Days Inns' September Days Club, and other senior organizations. Discounts vary depending on day or time of year.

DOLLAR—(800)421-6868. Dollar offers discounts to senior citizens 60 and over members of AARP.

HERTZ—(800) 654-3131. Hertz offers discounts to members of United Airlines' Silver Wings Plus Club, Days Inns' September Days Club, AARP, Y.E.S., and Mature Outlook.

NATIONAL—(800) 328-4567. National offers special discounts to members of Northwest Airlines' WorldHorizons Program, AARP, and Mature Outlook.

THRIFTY RENT-A-CAR—(800) 367-2277. Members of Northwest Airlines' WorldHorizons Program, AARP, CARP, Mature Outlook, and Days Inns' September Days Club are entitled to 10 percent senior discounts on car rentals worldwide. Thrifty, because of its association with AARP, has a unique program, "Give A Friend A Lift." For every 50,000 qualifying rentals made by members of AARP, Thrifty will donate a minivan for community services operated through Area Agencies on Aging. Area Agencies on Aging assist older Americans by providing services such as delivery of hot meals, chore services, energy assistance, adult day care, and transportation assistance.

TRAVELING WITH A GROUP: TOUR PROGRAMS

Tour programs come in many varieties from complete, door to door escorted excursions with everything planned and included, to highly individual programs where you are mostly on your own. Twenty-five years ago the idea of "taking a tour" meant taking a couple of weeks and covering several cities. Some companies still offer these breathless, whirlwind tours, but most are planned for a more relaxing, quality experience and are generally much less frantic. Your travel agent should recommend member tour operators of the NATIONAL TOUR ASSOCIATION (NTA), an organization requiring financial and performance standards of its members.

A tour package generally covers everything including most meals, transportation, escorts, sightseeing, group parties, etc. You are required to pay for the full tour in advance. Less-structured tours allow for individual travel activities, with airfare, hotel, airport transfers, and some meals, admissions, etc., included in the package. Since professional tour operators deal in large volume bookings at lower rates, the cost for a package tour is usually lower than if you were to pay for the elements separately.

To help you decide on a tour, make a list of your travel likes, dislikes, preferences, etc. Study brochure descriptions, which usually include details of daily itineraries and organized activities. This will aid you in choosing a tour that is right for you, either one that is strictly scheduled, loosely scheduled with lots of free time, or one somewhere in between.

Senior citizen discounts offered by tour operators vary by company, season, and other factors. As with all travel arrangements, ask your travel agent if there is a senior citizen discount for the tour you will be taking.

Some companies that focus their tour programs on mature travelers are:

YUGO TOURS—350 Fifth Ave., New York, NY 10118, (800) 223-5298, (212) 563-2400. This organization is owned by the Yugoslavian government. For those 49 or over, it offers its "Prime of Your Life Vacations" program, which has year-round trips to resorts of your choice in Yugoslavia. Rates very depending on the time of year, but all are very reasonable.

PLEASANT HAWAIIAN HOLIDAYS—2404 Townsgate Road, Westlake Village, CA 91361, (800) 242-9244. This company offers trips for those 60 or over to the Hawaiian Islands. Trips include flights, lodging (hotel or condo), side trips to other islands, breakfast, a rental car, transfers, counselors, a lei, and a memory album.

SENIOR TOURS INTERNATIONAL—P.O. Box 7404, Van Nuys, CA 91409, (818) 786-4321. This company specializes in affordable luxury tours for adults 50 and over. Groups of 20 or more are fully escorted by senior guides. There are more than 100 day tours and overnight trips to Las Vegas and Laughlin, Nevada, Lake Tahoe, San Diego, Big Bear, and other vacation/resort destinations covering Southern California.

SENIOR ESCORTED TOURS—223 N. Main Street, Cape May Court House, NJ 08210, (800) 222-1254. This tour group specializes in package trips to Cape May, New Jersey, the Catskill Mountains in New York, Nashville and Gatlinburg, Tenn., Cape Cod, Mass., and Orlando, Florida. Other vacations include cruises down the Mississippi River, through the Panama Canal, the coast of Alaska, in Australia, and visits to U.S. National Parks.

BREEZE TOURS—2750 Stickney Point Road, Sarasota, FL 33581, (800) 237-5630. Offers escorted sight-seeing trips to Hawaii, Australia, and New Zealand. Other trips for mature travelers include tours of British stately homes and castles and Hawaiian golfing tours.

TRAFALGAR'S AUTUMN YEARS TOURS—21 E. 26th St., New York, NY 10010, (800) 854-0103, (212) 689-8977. This British travel agency offers escorted motorcoach tours to those over 55. Most of the excursions are in Europe: England, Belgium, Holland, Germany, Austria, Switzerland, France, and Italy. Tour members are escorted by British tour directors.

TIPS FOR TRAVELING ABROAD

When traveling abroad for the first time, here are some important rules and suggestions to keep in mind.

Passports

Passports are required for entry into most foreign countries. Make sure yours is up to date; passports issued prior to 1982 are good for 8 years; passports issued after 1983 are good for 10 years. To apply for a passport contact your federal government building information center or the Passport Agency. Also, check with your local U.S. post office or local courthouse.

Apply for a passport two to three months prior to a planned trip, as it can take up to six weeks to process your application. You will need two photograph—one in color and one in black and white—to get your passport.

Currency

Get U.S. denomination travelers checks through your bank. Travelers checks are safer than cash, and if you don't use them, they can be used like money when you get home. Also, you won't have to pay an exchange fee to convert them back, like you do with foreign currency. Exchange most of you currency after you arrive since exchange rates are usually better in banks abroad. If you wish to exchange your dollars into foreign currencies before you leave, just exchange enough for incidentals like tips and taxis. Cash personal check only as you need them. Again, this will avoid having to exchange extra foreign currency back into dollars for a fee.

Vaccinations

In some areas of the world, particularly the tropics, you need certain vaccinations to protect your health. Ask your travel agent or call your state or local health department about required inoculations or vaccinations. Some medications and vaccinations must be taken two to four weeks in advance of travel, so check far enough ahead to be safe.

THE CENTER FOR DISEASE CONTROL in Atlanta has published a 10-page report on travel health precautions. Send $1 to: Sup. of Documents, Government Printing Office, Washington, D.C. 20402-9371. They also have a 24-hour hotline with international health requirements and health recommendations for foreign travelers. The number is (404) 332-4559.

Visas

Visas, similar to passports, are international identification cards. Ask you travel agent which countries require visas, or call the embassies of the countries you plan to visit. Visas are issued through the particular country's embassy in Washington, D.C., or the nearest consular office.

There are certain countries for which travel advisories are issued by the U.S. State Department because of uncertain or unsafe conditions for American travelers. The State Department maintains an Advisory Hotline, (202) 647-5225, which you can call for updated information.

Customs

You can bring up to $400 worth of new merchandise into the United States from abroad without paying taxes on it. The next $1,000 worth of goods is generally taxed at a 10 percent rate. The U.S. Customs Service publishes a free booklet "Know Before You Go," explaining all the customs procedures. For a copy write: Department of the Treasury, U.S. Customs Service, Washington, D.C. 20229.

The U.S. State Department has a brochure designed to alert Americans to potential risks of foreign travel and to raise security awareness. Topics include: how to contact American consulates or embassies in emergencies, how to obtain current travel advisories on hot spots around the world, and tips on medical matters, travel insurance, and visas. For a free copy write for: "What You Should Know Before You Go," Americans Abroad, Pueblo, CO 81009.

TRAVELING WITH THE GRANDKIDS

If you have grandchildren, traveling with them can be inexpensive, educational and can strengthen the bonds between you and your grandchildren. Many folks feel children between 7 and 13 travel best. They love to be in on the travel plans, helping to choose places to visit and things to see. As for saving money, airlines often offer discounts for children under 12 (as well as special companion fares) and most hotels allow them to stay in the same room with their grandparents at no extra charge. Cruise lines sometimes offer last-minute specials when they are underbooked, allowing kids to travel completely free. Travel with one of the groups below and not only see the world, but improve relationships and communication between generations.

EL AL'S GENERATION TO GENERATION TOURS—850 Third Avenue, New York, NY 10022, (800) 352-5786, (212) 486-2600. EL AL, the Israeli national airline, offers vacation opportunities for grandparents and grandchildren to Israel. Trips are planned so that visits to such places as Jerusalem, Tel Aviv, Masada, and the Dead Sea include special activities for both generations.

GRANDTRAVEL—6900 Wisconsin Avenue, Suite 706, Chevy Chase, Maryland 20815, (301) 986-0790, (800) 247-7651. This organization arranges tours for grandparents and grandchildren. GrandTravel's series of itineraries are scheduled for normal school breaks. They offer 15 tours, including travel to the western states and national parks, Washington, D.C., Alaska, Hawaii, an American Indian country tour, New England, the Soviet Union, Galapagos Islands, China and Japan, Africa, Scandinavia, Holland, England and Scotland, and New Zealand. Tours are developed by educators, psychologists, and leisure counselors and are structured to encompass both informational and recreational aspects. Trips focus on strengthening the bonds between the grandparent and grandchild, but there is plenty of time for everyone to be with people their own age.

MAYFLOWER TOURS—1225 Warren Avenue, P.O. Box 490, Downers Grove, Illinois 60515, (800) 323-7604, (708) 960-3430. Mayflower Tours offers special programs for senior citizens but does not have an age limit. Some senior travelers bring their grandchildren along on the tours. The minimum age for a child traveling on a Mayflower Tour is six years old.

RFD TRAVEL—4801 W. 110th St., Overland Park, KS 66211, (800)227-7737. RFD Travel organizes a summer American Heritage Tour that includes Philadelphia, Washington, D.C., Amish Pennsylvania, and Williamsburg. In winter they offer a California Rose Parade tour including San Diego and Anaheim.

SAGA HOLIDAYS—120 Boylston St., Boston, MA 02116, (800) 343-0273. Saga offers special tours for folks over 60 traveling with children between 6 and 16. Trips to scenic areas and places of interest in the Northwest, American Southwest, the California Coast and national parks are scheduled during regular school breaks.

THE TRAVELERS' SOCIETY—P.O. Box 2846, Loop Station, Minneapolis, MN 55402, (612) 342-2788. This is a non-profit organization whose objective is world peace and understanding of other peoples. They offer educational programs for grandparents and grandchildren with the purpose of providing opportunities for the two generations to share learning experiences about other cultures. There is a trip to the Soviet Union, a 10-day voyage to Kenya, visits to Ireland and England. Each trip offers its time for pleasure and relaxation, but all focus on learning about other cultures.

VISTATOURS—1923 N. Carson Street, Suite 105, Carson City, Nevada 89701, (800) 248-4782, (702) 882-2100. Vistatours offers a special tour series for grandparents and grandchildren. The tours schedule time for adults to be together with other adults at the same time the children are with other children. Grandparents and grandchildren also participate in activities together, giving the two generations the opportunity to share their traveling experiences.

ADVENTURES FOR THE
COURAGEOUS TRAVELER

If you have a spirited sense of adventure and lots of energy, consider traveling with one of these groups which specialize in challenging, exciting travel experiences.

AMERICAN WILDERNESS EXPERIENCE, A.W.E.—P.O. Box 1486, Boulder, Colorado 80306, (303) 494-2992, (800) 444-0099. American Wilderness Experience offers mature adults discounts on backcountry travel. Trips include a Bridger-Teton backcountry horseback trip in Wyoming, Sangre de Cristo Mountains horseback trip in Colorado, Mountain Sports Week Adventure in Colorado, a Colorado Surf and Turf Combo in Colorado, and an Alaska Wildlands Senior Safari Tour. In order to be eligible for the senior discounts you must be 65.

OUTWARD BOUND USA—384 Field Point Road, Greenwich, CT 06830, (800) 243-8520, (in Connecticut (203) 661-0797). The Outward Bound organization is well known for its wilderness-survival courses that are aimed to help youngsters and young adults. Mature adults can also discover new ways to go beyond their limitations through Outward Bound's shorter courses designed specifically for adults over 50. Some of the courses have a special goal of easing the transition from career to retirement.

Be prepared to live in a tent, sleep in sleeping bags, and cook your own food. Good health is a requirement to participate. Adventures include: courses in canoeing in the Florida Everglades, canoeing in the lake country of Minnesota, sailing in the Florida Keys, river rafting, desert backpacking or rock climbing on the West Coast, or white-river rafting, or hiking in North Carolina.

OVER THE HILL GANG—13791 E. Rice Pl., Aurora, CO 80015, (303) 699-6404. This organization is for people over 50 who are looking for action. Most of the trips are sports-oriented. Examples include ski trips to Vail, Colorado; Park City, Utah, and the Dolomites in Europe. There are cruises in the Caribbean and sightseeing vacations to Switzerland. To join your local Over the Hill Gang costs $50 or $80 per couple. There are over 1,000 members and 15 Gangs (chapters) coast to coast. If there is no local chapter in your area, you can join the national organization for $25 ($40 per couple) and participate in any of the organizations activities.

AMERICAN YOUTH HOSTELS—Dept. 855, P.O. Box 37613, Washington, D.C. 20013-7613, (202) 783-6161. This group coordinates more than 5,000 hostels in over 70 countries. If you want to go on an AYH trip anywhere in the world, you must be a member. Membership is $20 a year, but if you are 55, you only pay $10. AYH offers low-cost adventure trips for persons over 50 in its World Adventure trip program. Each trip is limited to 10 persons including a trip leader. You can tour all over the world by van, minibus, train, or bicycle. Some of their trips include: traveling by van to European cities; cycling in New England in the fall; a trip to the mountains, glaciers, and lakes of Alaska; five weeks by train and ferry through Europe; and hiking in the San Francisco Bay area.

BACKROADS BRITAIN—Campus Holidays USA, 242 Bellevue Ave., Upper Montclair, NJ 07043, (800) 526-2915. BB takes 12 people, age 50 and over, on "summertime only" two-week tours of the backroads of England, Scotland, and Wales, or Wales and Ireland. Groups are led by college professors. Accommodations include stays in country inns and bed and breakfasts, as well as traditional hotels.

CANADIAN HOSTELLING ASSOCIATION—333 River Road, Vanier, ON K1L 8H9, Canada, (613) 748-5638. Similar to the American Youth Hostel, the Canadian Hostelling Association offers adventures for all ages. There is no maximum age limit. As a member you can stay at a hostel for under $20 per night.

MT. ROBSON ADVENTURE HOLIDAY—P.O. Box 146, Valemount, BC V0E 2Z0, Canada, (604) 566-4351. This organization is designed specifically for travelers over 50. All of the trips are in Mount Washington Provincial Park located in the Canadian Rockies. Choose from helicopter camping trips, hiking trips, or trips canoeing in mountain lakes.

SENIOR TRAVEL EXCHANGE PROGRAM (STEP)—P.O. Box H, Santa Maria, CA 93456, (805) 925-5743. Like the student-exchange program, STEP promotes goodwill and world peace and is specifically for those over-50. You are matched with foreign hosts in countries of your choice, staying with families in private homes. STEP also offers vacations in low-cost resorts or inexpensive hotels. Send $3 for a brochure with trip details.

PEDAL POWER: BIKE TRAILS

If you are a serious biker, you may want to consider taking a trip along the 4,250 miles of the trans-America trail. This trail begins in Astoria, Oregon and goes to Yorkstown, Virginia, winding its way across country through small American towns. Campgrounds and inexpensive bike inns are situated along the way.

There are also several excellent companies that do nothing but plan biking tours and adventures. These companies offer trips all over the world for all levels of biking enthusiasts. Trips range from combination hiking/biking/backpacking vacations in Hawaii to luxury trips with gourmet meals and accommodations in four star French chateaux and English castles. Check with your travel agent for information and brochures.

NATIONAL PARKS AND GOVERNMENT RECREATION AREAS

Our national park system includes some of the most breathtaking, magnificent areas on this planet. These areas are maintained and preserved by the government for use by all people who wish to experience the breadth and depth of our precious natural resources and the richness of our cultural history. Travelers can enjoy educational, stimulating vacations visiting our national parks, national wildlife reserves, recreation areas, monuments, and historic sites. Some of these sites include: craters, swamps, seashores, caves, trading posts, battlefields, ships, military parks, historic homes, sand dunes, memorials, waterfalls, cliff dwellings, memorials, volcanoes, and giant redwood forests.

Information on national parks, historic sites, and monuments in the areas you plan to visit can be obtained free of charge by writing the NATIONAL PARK SERVICE, U.S. Department of the Interior, 18th & C Streets NW, Washington, D.C. 20240.

Since observing wildlife is a recreational hobby shared by many mature adults, you may want to visit one of the 450 National Wildlife Refuges that comprise over 90 million acres of lands and waters. Write to: DIVISION OF NATIONAL REFUGES, U.S. Fish and Wildlife Service, Department of the Interior, Washington, D.C. 20240, for brochures and information.

There are 156 national forests that stretch from Alaska to Puerto Rico that offer exciting opportunities for outdoor adventure. For a copy of the "National Forest Vacations," write: U.S. Department of Agriculture, Forest Service, Agriculture Building, 12th Street and Independence Avenue SW, P.O. Box 96090, Washington, D.C. 20090. Each regional office of the Forest Service has maps and literature about recreational facilities in the national forests. For information write: Regional Forester, USDA Forest Service at an area office of interest listed below:

ALASKA REGION
Federal Office Building
Box 1628
Juneau, AK 99801

EASTERN REGION
310 West Wisconsin Avenue
Milwaukee, WI 53203

INTERMOUNTAIN REGION
Federal Building
324-25th Street
Ogden, UT 84401

NORTHERN REGION
Federal Building
Missoula, MT 59807

PACIFIC NORTHWEST
 REGION
319 SW Pine Street
Portland, OR 97204

PACIFIC SOUTHWEST
 REGION
630 Sansome Street
San Francisco, CA 94111

ROCKY MOUNTAIN
 REGION
11177 W. 8th Avenue
Lakewood, CO 80215

SOUTHERN REGION
1720 Peachtree Avenue
Atlanta, GA 30309

SOUTHWESTERN REGION
517 Gold Avenue SW
Albuquerque, NM 87102

Some organizations offer wilderness trips in the national forests. Trips are organized with regard to differing levels of ability, with several designed with mature adults in mind. For information write:

APPALACHIAN MOUNTAIN   VERMONT HIKING
  CLUB   HOLIDAYS
5 Joy Street   P.O. Box 845
Boston, MA 02108   Waitsfield, VT 05673
(617) 523-0636   (802) 453-4816

SIERRA CLUB   THE WILDERNESS SOCIETY
730 Polk Street   1400 Eye Street
San Francisco, CA 94109   Washington, D.C. 20005
(415) 776-2211   (202) 833-2300

THE U.S. NATIONAL PARK SYSTEM

To obtain a list of all state tourism offices and their toll-free numbers send a self-addressed envelope to Discover America, Travel Industry Association of America, 2 Lafayette Center, 1133 21st St. NW, Washington, D.C. 20036. Or send for the "National Park Guide," National Park Service, U.S. Department of the Interior, 18th & C Streets NW, Washington, D.C. 20240.

THE GOLDEN AGE PASSPORT

The "Golden Age Passport" is a free lifetime permit to enter national parks, monuments, recreational areas, national wildlife refuges and historic sites. It is available to anyone over 62 and a permanent resident of the United States. "Golden Age Passports" must be obtained in person and proof of age (a driver's license, birth certificate or other identifying document) must be presented at a federally operated recreation area. Once issued the passport entitles you to receive 50 percent discounts on federal use fees for facilities and services such as camping, boat rentals, parking, cave tours, elevator services, etc. Also anybody accompanying a "Golden Age Passport" holder in a car or private vehicle also gets free admittance.

CHAPTER 5

HEALTH, WEALTH, AND WISE WAYS TO KEEP THEM

Finances and financial security—how to live within our means and finding safe ways to invest our money—are major concerns for mature adults. In our "earning years," making money is our primary concern. As we approach retirement, keeping it becomes our main focus.

Retirement plans abound. There are seemingly endless numbers of investment firms, brokers, and counselors who would like to help you invest your money for retirement (which, of course, generates fees and commissions for them). Although there are many different types of plans available, we are going to look at how to get the best free and low-cost retirement/savings investment advice and where to find special savings available only to mature adults.

Along with money, the cost of health care is a major concern of seniors. Health care costs are expected to continue to increase more than 10 percent a year over the next several years. The subjects of funding for Medicare, HMOs, supplemental insurance plans, and planning for long-term care are topics that are constantly being debated by our local, state, and national representatives. We are going to examine both how to obtain free health care (when available) and how to find the most cost effective health care benefits and programs. As complex as these issues seem, there are sources of information to help us better understand them.

FREE PROGRAMS AND SERVICES FROM YOUR BANK

With banks and savings and loans in fierce competition for your funds, there has emerged a whole area of privileges, perks, and special programs for seniors. It is estimated that some 63 million Americans age 50 and older hold approximately two thirds of all bank savings deposits and approximately 80 percent of savings and loan deposits. This group, expected to grow by 14 million in the next 10 years, has a median net worth almost double that for the population as a whole—$60,226. It's not difficult to understand why banks and S&Ls are literally fighting for these funds. In most cases the rate of investment return is virtually the same among competing institutions, so they have come up with all kinds of ways to entice us into saving. This translates into free benefits for seniors including:

- Free checking accounts;
- Free safe deposit boxes;
- Free photocopying;
- Added percentage points on invested funds;
- Free checks;
- Free notary service;
- Free telephone and wire service transfers;
- Free traveler's checks, cashier's checks and money orders;
- Newsletters;
- Waiver of service charges on bank card membership;
- Overdraft protection on checking accounts;
- Seminars on tax-free investing, health, and fitness;
- Free subscriptions to senior publications;
- Travel discounts;
- Membership in dining clubs;

- Discounts on merchandise, entertainment, dental care, vitamins, eyewear, automobiles.

These are some of the "extras" banks offer seniors and preferred customers to gain their business and lasting loyalty. Once you open an account or buy a CD, these banks are hoping you'll become interested in their trust services, home-equity loans, reverse mortgages, etc.

The concept of free senior services began 15 years ago when Santa Barbara Bank and Trust Company set up their successful Our Gang program. Below are examples of financial institutions around the country that currently offer senior savings clubs and service programs:

CITISENIORS, Citibank Maryland; FLORIDIAN CLUB, Citizens and Southern National Bank of Florida; CLUB 50, Meridian Bank of Reading, Pennsylvania; SENIOR PARTNERS, Barnett Bank in Jacksonville, Florida; PORTFOLIO 50, Bank of Boston; PRIME ADVANTAGE, Society Bank; AMERICAN PATRIOTS CLUB, American Savings Bank, locations throughout California; FIFTY PLUS CHECKING, Fortune Savings Bank, locations in Florida; SENIOR ADVANTAGE, Great American Bank, locations in Arizona, Washington, and Montana.

To find out more information about the above programs, contact directory assistance for a toll-free number for the one(s) located in your state. Or call your bank or savings and loan and ask whether they have a special program for senior customers.

As in other industries, senior discounts and services are not always advertised or disclosed at first glance. You need to inquire as to what you can get just because you are a mature adult. Make a list of the kinds of "extra" services you feel are important and present them to the bank officer responsible for new accounts. They may just offer you what you want. When deciding where to entrust your funds, compare requirements for maintaining minimum balances, service charges, and interest rates.

TAX RELIEF

If you need information or help with your taxes, the IRS offers free publications on a large number of tax topics. In fact, there is an IRS publication that covers just about every item that appears on a Form

1040. Although these publications go into great detail, they are written simply and accurately. There is even a publication that contains a list of all the other free publications entitled: "Guide to Free Tax Services." You can receive these publications by (l) calling the IRS's toll-free number (800) 424-FORM; (2) going to your local IRS office, post office, bank, or library and seeing whether their supply of bulletins includes what you are looking for; or (3) writing the Forms Distribution Center for your state (the address is listed in the Form 1040 booklet).

The IRS also has a toll-free volunteer telephone tax assistance number for specific questions on filling out your forms. This service, called Volunteers In Tax Assistance (VITA), works best for those with simple returns. The number is: (800) TAX-1040. For more complex tax returns, a professional tax preparer, tax service, or accountant is recommended.

In addition, the AARP has over 8,000 Tax-Aide service sites manned by volunteer tax counselors who help low- and moderate-income tax-payers over 60 with filing their income tax returns. For information call your local AARP chapter.

RETIREMENT RECOMMENDATIONS

There are several sources of free and low cost information and advice on how to prepare for retirement. The Administration on Aging publishes booklets covering retirement topics including:

"Every Tenth American," describing the programs of the Administration on Aging;

"Are You Planning on Living the Rest of Your Life?" a do-it-yourself planner for people without preretirement counseling services provided by their jobs;

"You, the Law and Retirement," which explains when and why to see a lawyer;

"Consumer Guide for Older People," a wallet-size folder that outlines ways older folks can protect themselves against rip-offs, frauds, and swindlers.

To receive any of the booklets on the previous page, write: U.S. DEPT. OF HEALTH AND HUMAN SERVICES, COMMISSIONER ON AGING, 200 Independence Ave., S.W., Washington, D.C. 20201.

IDS FINANCIAL SERVICES has a free booklet entitled "What Do I Want to Be...When I Retire? Financial Planning for Retirement," which exlpains how much money you will need to retire and ways to minimize taxes, update your will and check your health insurance. It also lists groups that can help. They also publish a free 20-page guide, "Financial Planning: How It Works For You." For either publication write: IDS Consumer Affairs, IDS Financial Services, Inc., IDS Tower 10, Minneapolis, MN 55440.

Another source of information available through COMMERCE CLEARING HOUSE is "On Your Retirement: Tax and Benefit Considerations." This booklet discusses Social Security and Medicare benefits, private pensions and annuities, IRAs, and tax breaks available to older Americans. Copies are $5, plus tax, handling and shipping. Write: Commerce Clearing House, Inc. 4025 W. Peterson Ave., Chicago, IL 60646 or call them toll-free at (800) 248-3248.

JOHN HANCOCK FINANCIAL SERVICES will send you a free "Retirement Planning Guide" showing you how much money you'll need for a comfortable retirement. Write to: John Hancock Mutual Funds, 101 Huntington Avenue, Boston, MA 02199-7603.

THE ARTHRITIS FOUNDATION's Planned Giving Committee organizes volunteer attorneys and financial planners who speak on such topics as estate planning, financial planning, and tax planning. These seminars and workshops are offered free to the general public. Contact your local chapter of the Arthritis Foundation for a copy of the calendar of programs in your area.

THE NEW ENGLAND MUTUAL LIFE INSURANCE COMPANY has prepared a free guide "How to Prepare for a Financially Secure Retirement." For a copy write: The New England, 501 Boylston St., Boston, MA 02117.

One of the best resources on retirement is the *United Retirement Bulletin*. A year's subscription costs $29. For a free sample issue, send a SASE to: Edith Tucker, Editor, United Retirement Bulletin, 210 Newbury St., Boston, MA 02116.

Another recommended newsletter is *The Retirement Letter*, edited by Peter A. Dickinson, author of several books on retirement. A year's subscription is $87, but you can receive a free sample issue by enclosing a SASE to: Peter A. Dickinson, The Retirement Letter, 44 Wildwood Drive, Prescott, AZ 86301.

The Mature Investor is a newsletter edited by J. Kevin Donovan, a Certified Financial Planner, offering investment advice in several areas including mutual funds, CDs, Treasuries, money market funds, and stocks. A regular one-year subscription is $99 or you can get a special six-month trial subscription for $29.95. For information write: The Mature Investor, OXO Publishing Inc., P.O. Box 2741, Glen Ellyn, IL 60139-9954; or call (800) 678-8537.

The Preston Report is a bimonthly retirement planning newsletter edited by Robert Preston. For subscription information write: 57 North St., Danbury, CT 06810.

Your financial planner, accountant, insurance agent, or securities broker should be able to advise you on your choices of investment vehicles for safeguarding your money and insuring income for you and your family's future. Mutual funds, stock funds, bond funds, CDs, money market funds, tax-free income funds, taxable-income funds, growth-income funds, fixed-income funds, IRAs, Keoughs, annuities, reverse mortgages, living trusts, 401(k) plans, etc., are just some of the investment alternatives and opportunities available in today's complex financial marketplace.

In case you are confused by these terms, here are a few simple definitions to help you:

Annuity: A life-insurer's contract whose earnings are tax deferred. The income from an annuity can be paid out over a lifetime, both yours and your spouse's, or over a certain number of years.

Defined contribution plan: A company savings plan in which earnings on investments are tax deferred until they are withdrawn. Employees, employers, or both can contribute to these plans.

401(k) plan: A type of defined-contribution plan also known as a salary-reduction plan. An employee puts a certain percentage of annual pretax salary into a 401(k), and the earnings grow tax-deferred until withdrawn.

Individual retirement account (IRA): A tax-deferred savings plan available to anyone who earns money. Depending on your income and whether you or your spouse is covered by a pension plan, the contributions to an IRA may be tax deductible.

Keogh plan: For people who are self-employed, this retirement savings plan offers contributions that are tax-deductible and earnings that are tax-deferred until withdrawn.

Reverse mortgage: This is a loan designed for retired people. It pays a homeowner a fixed monthly amount and defers repayment of principal and interest until the home is sold. (For more information on this subject write for AARP's free booklet, "Home Made Money," AARP-HEIC, 1909 K St., N.W., Washington, D.C. 20049.)

Retirement and estate planning are gaining more importance and recognition as people continue to live longer, fuller, and more active lives. If you do not have a trusted financial advisor, ask your friends or business associates to recommend one. Or contact one of the following national organizations for help in finding a qualified financial planner in your area:

INSTITUTE FOR CERTIFIED FINANCIAL PLANNERS
10065 East Harvard Avenue
Denver, CO 80231
(303) 751-7600

INTERNATIONAL ASSOCIATION OF FINANCIAL PLANNING
Registry of Financial Planning Practitioners
2 Concourse Parkway #800
Atlanta, GA 30328
(404) 395-1605

NATIONAL ASSOCIATION OF PERSONAL FINANCIAL
  ADVISORS (fee-only planners)
(312)-537-7722

If you are looking for a stockbroker, choose one whose firm is registered with the SEC. The broker must personally be registered with the National Association of Securities Dealers. If you want to check whether there have been any security-related disciplinary actions, contact your state securities commission. (You can get the number through the North American Securities Administrators Association Hotline: (800) 942-9022). Or you can file a public disclosure form with the NATIONAL ASSOCIATION OF SECURITIES DEALERS, 9514 Key West Ave., Rockville, MD 20850, (301) 590-6500. Always get an independent second opinion, or investigate yourself before investing.

If you are using a professional money manager, they must be registered with the SEC. The Freedom of Information Branch of the SEC (202-272-7440) or your state securities commission can check their records for you.

A professional insurance agent should be a C.L.U., meaning chartered life underwriter or C.P.C.U., chartered property/casualty underwriter. Your state insurance commission (the number is in the state government listing section of your phone book) can give you records of disbarment.

For preparing taxes and other financial services, a professional accountant should be a certified public accountant (C.P.A.), licensed by the state. The state board of accountancy (the number is among the state government listings in the phone book) will let you know if any disciplinary or licensing actions have been brought forth.

For advice on buying, selling, or investing in real estate, work with a real estate broker or sales agent who is licensed by the state. They should also be a member of the National Association of Realtors® or the local board of Realtors®. Your state real estate commission (again, the number is in the state government listings in the phone book) can alert you to any past problems. Unless you know your agent well, similar to our advice regarding stock brokers, investigate and get independent advice before buying.

Another interesting and free source of information on investing for retirement can be found in the columns and features of senior magazines and newspapers. Most publications have a regular section on personal finance and/or money matters. A variety of questions pertaining to seniors is addressed in these pages. Their in-depth articles can help clarify and explain a lot of the confusion regarding money and investments. Most of these publications are subscribed to by local libraries and senior citizen centers. They are also distributed free in markets and some restaurants.

WHERE TO GO FOR ANSWERS ON MEDICARE AND INSURANCE

You will probably qualify for Medicare at age 65, but the program currently only covers little more than a third of actual medical costs. Chances are you will need either a medical supplement policy or an all-inclusive HMO or health insurance program to add to or replace Medicare. Medicare was never intended to be an all-inclusive health insurance program, and these supplemental policies offer coverage and benefits not covered by Medicare.

Trying to make sense of the several health coverage options that are available can be difficult and confusing; however, there are sources of information and education to help you understand these options.

"A Consumer's Guide to Long-Term Care Insurance" and "Health Care and Finances: A Guide for Adult Children and Their Parents," are available for $.50 each through the CONSUMER INFORMATION CATALOG, Consumer Information Center-N, P.O. Box 100, Pueblo, CO 81002.

The SENIOR CITIZENS HEALTH INSURANCE COUNSELING program (SCHIC) is a free service provided by THE NATIONAL ASSOCIATION OF LIFE UNDERWRITERS, which helps seniors evaluate their health care needs and educates them about fraudulent insurance schemes and solicitations. Active or retired insurance agents in more than twenty states participate in the program. For information write: The National Association of Life Underwriters, 1922 F St., N.W., Washington, D.C. 20006-4387.

THE HEALTH INSURANCE ASSOCIATION OF AMERICA, P.O. Box 41455, Washington, D.C. 20018, Tel: (201) 223-7780, has two excellent free pamphlets entitled: "The Consumer's Guide to Medicare Supplement Insurance" and "The Consumer's Guide to Long-Term Care Insurance."

In California, the Department of Insurance has a free six-page protection kit for seniors concerning Medicare supplement insurance. The kit is available through the office of Paul A. Woodruff, Assemblyman, San Bernardino County, 300 E. State Street, #480, Redlands, CA 92373.

Also in California, the HEALTH INSURANCE COUNSELING AND ADVOCACY PROGRAM (HICAP) of the California Dept. of Aging and the Legal Services Trust Fund organizes free educational programs and seminars on Medicare and HMOs through its Medicare Advocacy Project (MAP). MAP is an independent, nonprofit organization not affiliated with Medicare or any insurance company or Health Maintenance Organization. Senior citizen clubs, community centers, hospitals, medical centers and related organizations can schedule one of their specialists for a presentation. Some of the topics covered include: Nuts and Bolts of Medicare; Who Pays for Skilled Nursing and Long-Term Care?; Filling the Medicare Gaps: What Supplemental Insurance Can Do; What You Should Know Before Joining An HMO. For information on their programs telephone (800) 824-0780.

Most hospitals and medical centers also sponsor their own free seminars on investment management needs, health care, and life insurance. These are usually coordinated through their senior or geriatric health departments and are advertised in local newspapers, senior publications, and mailings. Check with the hospitals in your area for a schedule of upcoming seminars.

In addition, some of the large federally qualified health plan organizations sponsor lectures and presentations throughout the year at various locations. Their schedules are usually advertised in local senior publications and magazines. Two examples are SECUREHORIZONS and SENIOR PLAN FHP HEALTH CARE.

Senior newspapers and magazines, along with their recommendations on investment and money matters, offer a wealth of interesting and informative advice in all areas of health care and insurance. Nearly every publication has a regular feature or column answering readers' questions on these subjects. These "health" columnists and editors are specialists in their field and offer consumers sound advice and referrals for additional information. These publications also feature monthly calendar listings of dozens of free lectures, screenings, health fairs and expos, flu shot clinics, etc. By taking advantage of these free community services, you can save yourself a lot of money on what is generally routine, preventive health care that costs a lot more with a private practitioner.

Some insurance companies offer discounts on automobile insurance rates for seniors, who incidentally have better driving records than other age groups. Most independent agents represent at least one company offering special senior rates. Examples of insurance companies that give "senior rates" for good drivers include: STATE FARM INSURANCE COMPANY, NATIONWIDE INSURANCE, LIBERTY MUTUAL INSURANCE GROUP, and ALLSTATE INSURANCE COMPANY. The AARP also has an automobile insurance program, and several of the national senior organizations offer insurance discounts with membership. Your automobile club may also offer special discounts to their senior members who drive. Check with the individual organizations for their benefits.

CHAPTER 6

YOU'RE NEVER TOO OLD TO LEARN

Education is a lifetime process. Now, for the first time in many of our lives, we can choose to learn about the things we really want to know. Our choices cover a wide spectrum, from regular graded classes and curriculum to special classes offered specifically for mature adults. As seniors, we make the decisions on where to study, what to study, and how much or how hard to study. Now is the time to expand your horizons and learn for your own personal enjoyment and growth. School was never like this back when we were kids!

Practically every institution in the United States and Canada welcomes older adults into its regular programs, with a large majority offering reduced tuition and fees. If you wish to take courses for credit towards earning a degree or diploma, you may do so. However, if you simply wish to add to your knowledge, most schools will allow you to audit or monitor their classes.

In addition to the education you are receiving, going back to school is a wonderful opportunity to increase your social contacts and make friends. In fact, younger students actually benefit from working alongside mature adults and gaining special insights from their life experiences and knowledge of the "real" world. At the same time, those returning to school, even after several decades away from the classroom, have been found to more than hold their own in courses with younger students.

LEARNING CENTERS:
A NEW TWIST TO ADULT EDUCATION

A recent development in adult education that has gained popularity is the formation of adult learning centers offering a wide variety of short-term, practical, high-quality courses at reasonable fees. Most courses cost between $25 and $50 (except computer courses, which are usually under $100). Classes are taught by consultants, entrepreneurs, business owners, professionals, medical professionals, etc., who enjoy teaching adults in the community.

Programs center around topics such as finding new and unusual careers, improving relationships, self-improvement, real estate, hands-on computer literacy, money management, creative and career writing, hobbies, sports and recreation, entertaining, cooking, and other "non-traditional" topics. Classes generally meet once a week in the evenings. There are no grades, no exams, and no degrees. These programs are strictly for those who want to expand their knowledge in interesting, practical, and fun areas.

THE LEARNING ANNEX is a national franchise with centers located in Los Angeles, San Diego, San Francisco, New York, Washington, D.C., and Toronto. Since it first began 10 years ago, 1.3 million students have attended more than 132,000 Learning Annex classes. For information on Learning Annex courses contact: The Learning Annex, Corporate Office, 2330 Broadway, New York, NY 10024 or call the Learning Annex in one of the above cities.

Below are names and phone numbers of other adult learning centers around the country offering similar programs:

BOSTON CENTER FOR ADULT EDUCATION, Boston, Massachusetts, (617) 267-4430.

DISCOVERY CENTER, Chicago, Illinois, (312) 348-8120.

DISCOVERY CENTER, Cincinnati, Ohio, (512) 221-6800.

DISCOVERY CENTER, New York, New York, (800) 777-0338.

FIRST CLASS, Washington, D.C., (202) 797-5102.

THE INFORMATION EXCHANGE, Los Angeles, California, (213) 388-2800.

THE INFORMATION NETWORK, Pasadena, California, (818) 441-4080.

THE LEARNING CONNECTION, Providence, Rhode Island, (401) 247-9330.

MT. AIRY LEARNING TREE, Philadelphia, Pennsylvania, (215) 849-5500.

OPEN U, Minneapolis, Minnesota, (612) 379-3846.

TRAVEL AND LEARN

Mature adults are among the largest percentage of national and international travelers. They also enjoy learning while they travel. As a result there are several extensive college campus and learning programs worldwide tailored as learning experiences for seniors.

Elderhostel

Last year over 190,000 people filled classrooms all over the United States and around the world through ELDERHOSTEL, a nonprofit organization with the philosophy that education can be fulfilling and fun. Elderhostel has one- and two-week programs at more than 1,200 colleges, universities, research stations, and other educational institutions around the globe. Each offers low-cost sessions for people 60 years and older.

Classes are a blend of lectures, cultural events, local exploration, and social activity. They cover such diverse subjects as local history and culture, archaeology, the sciences, arts, and literature. The Elderhostel catalog is produced seasonally and filled with fascinating, enticing programs. We discovered the catalog at our local library and spent several hours poring over its wonderful courses.

The cost of Elderhostel is intentionally held to modest levels, consistent with traditional hosteling philosophy. Accommodations are simple and the food wholesome and nutritious. The typical charge for an all-inclusive six-night program in the United States is $255; in Canada $275. For a free catalog write: Elderhostel, 80 Boyle Street, Suite 400, Boston, MA 02116.

Interhostel

Interhostel is an international study-travel program for energetic people over 50. Sponsored by the University of New Hampshire, Interhostel offers two-week "educational experiences" at colleges and universities in Europe, China, and Australia. Programs combine lessons in history and culture with lectures, field trips, and social activities.

As with the Elderhostel program, costs are kept moderate. Included are two weeks' full room and board, tuition, and ground transportation. For information write: Interhostel, University of New Hampshire, 6 Garrison Ave., Durham, NH 03824; (800) 733-9753.

UNIVAC

The UNIVAC (University Vacations) program has summer sessions from one to twelve weeks at either Oxford or Cambridge Universities in England. University scholars engage students with morning lectures in English history, literature, and culture. Afternoons are dedicated to tours, excursions, and side trips. For information contact: Oxford-Cambridge Univac, 9602 N.W. 13th Street, Miami, FL 33172.

International Friendship Service

This is a low-cost program offering intensive instruction in a foreign language at a European university. Study programs range from two to five weeks and are offered at different times throughout the year. Concentrated instruction in French, Spanish, or Italian is given at universities in Neuchatel, Switzerland; Malaga, Spain; Cannes or Paris, France; Florence,Italy; and the island of Corsica.

The moderately priced packages include simple lodging, some meals, excursions, and tuition. School activities include lectures by guest speakers, concerts, sports, and parties. For more information write: International Friendship Service, 22994 El Toro Rd., El Toro, CA 92630.

Northeastern Senior Seminars

These are a series of one-week summer residential seminars given at several New York universities. You must be 55 or older to be eligible for the programs. A wide range of courses is offered along with side trips to places of interest in the surrounding areas. Participants live in dorms and are given three meals a day for approximately $300 per week. There are also commuter rates. Contact: Summer Special Programs, Skidmore College, Saratoga Springs, NY 12866 for information.

Senior Ventures

Sponsored by Central Washington University, this program offers two- and four-week SENIOR VENTURES sessions. Seniors participate in in-class learning, class-related excursions, and just-for-the-fun-of-it explorations of Washington State. For information: Senior Ventures, Central Washington University, Ellensburg, WA 98926, (800) 752-4380.

Language Study Abroad

The Senior Study Center division of this organization offers vacation/holiday packages combined with in-depth language instruction. A recent fully-escorted tour to Cuernavaca, Mexico included daily three-hour classes in Spanish. There are optional social and cultural activities with excursions to nearby historical and archaeological sites, villages and a typical Indian market.

They also offer similar programs in Spanish in Seville, Spain, and in French in Vichy, France. For information on tours write: Senior Study Center—Language Study Abroad, 1301 N. Maryland Ave., Glendale, CA 91207.

For a full range of adult study-vacation programs, the first edition of *The Guide to Academic Travel* describes programs for people of all ages offered by 258 colleges and universities, museums and historical societies, nature and environmental organizations, and travel companies. Included in the 240-page guide is a list of 93 sponsors whose programs offer an environmental or ecological focus. The guide can be found in most public libraries and bookstores, or it can be ordered for $16.95 from

Shaw Associates, 625 Biltmore Way, Coral Gables, FL 33134, (305) 446-8888.

Travel and Learn: The New Guide to Educational Travel is another book that provides detailed information on more than a thousand educational travel programs in the United States and abroad, including archaeology and history trips, music workshops, museum tours, art courses, cultural seminars for studying business abroad, language programs, outdoor and ecology programs. Single copies are $26 (including shipping). Order from: Blue Penguin Publications, 147 Sylvan Ave., Leonia, NJ 07605.

Workshops Around the World is a series of practical guides describing worldwide courses, conferences, and workshops on cooking, writing, photography, arts and crafts, the arts, humanities, sciences, and nature. They are $16.95 each and can be ordered through the Book Passage catalog, (800) 321-9785. *Work, Study & Travel Abroad* is an excellent basic sourcebook for travel adventurers of any age. It introduces opportunities for inexpensive travel, government grants, scholarships, volunteer and exchange programs, teaching, interns, etc. It costs $10.95 and is also available through Book Passage.

GO TO THE HEAD OF THE CLASS

North Carolina Center for Creative Retirement

The purpose of the center is to help enrich the lives of retirement-age people and, in fact, benefit Americans of all generations through educational and cultural programs. Eight programs are offered for those over 50 looking for ways to build fulfilling lives for themselves and others. The programs include: Senior Leadership Seminars in history, culture, politics, economics, and social structure; the Retirement Wellness Center for training seniors to be wellness advocates in their community; The College for Seniors, where classes are free from the pressures of testing and grades; Retirement Issues Forum; The Research Institute; the Retirement Planning Program; and The Senior Academy for Intergenerational Learning, where retired experts work with undergraduates. Contact: The North Carolina Center for Creative Retirement, Owen Hall, UNC Asheville, Asheville, NC 28804-3299.

Close Up Foundation

For those 50 and older the Program for Older Americans provides up close, behind-the-scenes educational tours of Washington, D.C., and other places. The purpose is to give individuals a first-hand look at how government functions in our capital city. Activities include walks on Capitol Hill, seminars with key Washington personalities, bus tours, workshops and briefings on current events and issues, and social activities. These one-week programs give seniors a great opportunity to enhance their knowledge about our country's political process. Contact: CLOSE UP FOUNDATION, Program for Older Americans, 1235 Jefferson Davis Highway, Arlington, VA 22202, (800) 232-2000.

University Seniors

New York University offers people over 65 two free university courses per semester and biweekly luncheon discussions on current events and topics of interest. Contact: University Seniors, NYU School of Continuing Education, 11 W. 42nd St., New York, NY 10036.

"Go-60" Program

Pennsylvania State University will give college credit courses at half tuition for seniors over 60 who are retired or employed less than half-time and are current residents of Pennsylvania, former Penn State students, or former Penn State employees. Contact: Independent Learning Office, Pennsylvania State University, 128 Mitchell Building, University Park, PA, 16802, (800) 458-3617; (800)252-3592 (in PA).

The Smithsonian Institution

The Resident Associate Program (RAP), a privately supported membership arm of THE SMITHSONIAN INSTITUTION, presents a wide variety of enriching education opportunities including cultural activities and public outreach programs. Resident members receive advance notice of programs and significantly reduced admittance fees for performing arts programs, lectures, films, seminars, studio arts, and courses. Contact the Resident Associate Program, The Smithsonian Institution, Washington, D.C. 20560.

Chautauqua Institution

This institution sponsors summer weekends and one-week programs for folks over 55 at an 856-acre site on the shore of Lake Chautauqua, New York. A wide variety of educational programs with discussions, workshops, lectures, films, evening entertainment, and recreational activities are offered at this relatively inexpensive adult summer camp. Fees cover tuition, room, meals, and activities. For information write: Helen Overs, Program Center of Older Adults, Chautauqua, NY 14722.

The College at 60 - New York City

The Lincoln Center campus of Fordham University offers credit college courses in liberal arts subjects taught by Fordham faculty members. Actually available to adults over 50, the program includes a lecture series and use of all campus facilities. Contact: The College at 60, Fordham University at Lincoln Center, 113 W. 60th St., New York, NY 10023.

Duquesne University

Duquesne University offers senior citizens over 60 discounts for full- or part-time study for one degree. For information write: Duquesne University, Office of Admissions, Pittsburgh, PA 15282.

The Educational Network for Older Adults

A network of 65 colleges and universities, adult organizations, community centers, and associations in Chicago whose purpose is to help older people find educational and training programs. The ENOA Resource Center offers free information on vocational programs, job assistance programs, educational programs, financial-retirement seminars, business opportunities for older adults, etc. Contact: THE EDUCATION NETWORK FOR OLDER ADULTS, 36 S. Wabash, Suite 624, Chicago, IL 60603.

Elder College at Hofstra

Located in Hempstead, New York, this is a series of one-week (Mon-Fri.) commuter programs for people over 60 covering a variety of cultural and historical subjects. For information write: Elder College at Hofstra, UCCE, 232 Memorial Hall, Hempstead, NY 11550.

SENIORNET

SeniorNet is a nonprofit organization whose purpose is to bring information-age technologies to adults over 55 by teaching computer skills. This program originated at the University of San Francisco as a research project to study the use of computer communication networking by older adults. Members throughout the United States and Canada communicate with one another and gain access to information of interest to them. SeniorNet currently sponsors 32 sites around the country for training, networking, and sociability. They also offer computer classes designed especially for older adults. There are more than 3,500 SeniorNet members linked by a national on-line computer network. Membership includes a quarterly newsletter, discounts on hardware and software products, a discounted registration to the annual SeniorNet conference, and a copy of the book, *Computers for Kids over Sixty*. Members pay a one-time fee of $15 to set up a network account (monthly subscription fees and hourly rates are extra). For information contact: SeniorNet, 399 Arguello Blvd., San Francisco, CA 94118.

HIGHER EDUCATION
WITHOUT THE STRESS

There are several programs throughout the country affiliated with colleges, universities, and learning institutes that offer senior or adult-oriented stress-free (no grades, no tests) classes. The courses are led by professionals who offer their expertise on a wide variety of subjects. Students pay an annual fee to the sponsoring university and may take as many courses as they wish (some also charge a reduced fee for individual courses). Included are campus privileges and use of campus facilities. Contact the individual campuses listed below for details of their programs:

ACADEMY OF LIFELONG LEARNING, University of Delaware, 2800 Pennsylvania Ave., CED, Wilmington, DE 19806.

CENTER FOR CREATIVE RETIREMENT, Long Island University, Southampton, NY 11968-4198.

CENTER FOR LEARNING IN RETIREMENT, University of California Extension Center, 55 Laguna St., San Francisco, CA 94102.

EDUCATIONAL GROWTH OPPORTUNITIES (EGO), College of Extended Studies, San Diego State University, 4075 Park Blvd., San Diego, CA 92103.

THE HARVARD INSTITUTE FOR LEARNING IN RETIREMENT, Lehman Hall B-3, Cambridge, MA 02138.

THE INSTITUTE FOR LEARNING IN RETIREMENT, American University, Nebraska Hall, 4400 Massachusetts Ave. N.W., Washington, D.C. 20016.

INSTITUTE FOR RETIRED PROFESSIONALS, New School for Social Research, 66 W. 12th St., New York, NY 10011.

INSTITUTE OF NEW DIMENSIONS, Palm Beach Junior College, 3160 PGA Blvd., Palm Beach Gardens, FL 33410.

LEARNING IN RETIREMENT, Duke University, Durham, NC 27708.

NOVA COLLEGE INSTITUTE FOR RETIRED PROFESSIONALS, 3301 College Ave., Fort Lauderdale, FL 33314.

THE PLATO SOCIETY OF UCLA, University of California at Los Angeles, 10995 Le Conte Ave., Los Angeles, CA 90024.

PROFESSIONALS AND EXECUTIVES IN RETIREMENT, Hofstra University, 1000 Hempstead Turnpike, Hempstead, NY 11550.

TEMPLE ASSOCIATION FOR RETIRED PROFESSIONALS (TARP), Temple University Center City Campus, 1616 Walnut Street, Room 600, Philadelphia, PA 19103.

CHAPTER 7

HERE'S TO YOUR HEALTH AND KEEPING IT

No one will argue that over 50, our bodies begin to go through a lot of changes. These changes are as normal and natural as anything else in our lives. At the same time, remaining strong, fit, and healthy after 50 will allow us to enjoy all the wonderful benefits that are available to us. This chapter will give you the sources of information and preventive care to help maintain the highest quality of health, your most precious commodity, throughout your life.

Since maintaining and improving health is such an important, universal concern, many dedicated individuals, groups, and nonprofit organizations offer free or low-cost testing, screening, and information on a variety of health concerns specifically related to the needs of older Americans.

Even with Medicare, Medicaid, and the numerous supplemental medical insurance plans, costs for preventive tests and exams are not always affordable. However, there are public and private facilities that offer screenings, health assessments, and health education sessions as a public service. Look for advertisements for these screenings and health checks in the women's or life-style section of your local newspaper. Some hospitals and medical facilities send out mailings announcing times and dates of free medical testing for seniors. Check senior newspapers for calendar listings and ads on upcoming testing dates. (These newspapers are often distributed free in markets, restaurants, libraries, and drugstores.)

Many national associations, organizations, foundations, and manufacturers of medical equipment designate certain times of the year as "National _____ Prevention Month." For example, May is Better Hearing and Speech Month, September is National Breast Cancer

Month, Adult Immunization Week comes at the end of October, and there is an Osteoporosis Prevention Week. During these designated weeks and months, vigorous campaigns and programs are implemented nationwide to create awareness of techniques of early testing and treatment for practically every illness from the flu to breast cancer.

Announcements of free and low-cost clinics associated with these yearly campaigns are usually made through local newspapers and publications.

Some companies use their medical departments or work with community agencies and local hospitals to provide a wide variety of screenings to determine employees' risk for developing certain diseases. Blood pressure screenings are the most common, but more comprehensive testing of blood and cholesterol levels are becoming available. Some companies will even provide follow up sessions with company doctors. This form of preventative care saves thousands of dollars in anticipated medical costs to companies offering medical insurance and coverage to employees.

In addition, there are many companies and manufacturers in the medical equipment and pharmaceutical fields that offer mobile testing services at local pharmacies, markets, shopping malls, health fairs, and health expos. Screenings include vision and hearing exams, podiatric exams, diabetic and glucose tolerance tests, mammograms, general dental screenings, body composition, pulmonary function tests, blood pressure, cholesterol, and stroke detection tests.

WHERE TO FIND BOOKS AND INFORMATION ON HEALTH

The NATIONAL INSTITUTE ON AGING offers free publications covering many areas of health and aging. Some of their titles include:

Accidental Hypothermia; Exercise Packet; Nutrition Packet; Resource Directory for Older People; The Menopause Time of Life; What Is Your Aging IQ?; Women's Age Page Packet.

Of special interest to women is the guide entitled "Health Resources for Older Women," a 75-page booklet that describes the normal changes that take place during the aging process as well as conditions like arthritis and osteoporosis that become more prevalent in later years. The booklet provides a useful introduction to the challenges that mature women face (including financial planning, caregiving, housing options, and widowhood) and offers good tips on ways to deal with them.

The NIA also publishes a series called "Age Pages," which provide a quick, practical look at health topics that interest older people. There are over forty "Age Pages" covering the following areas:

Diseases and Disorders; Health Promotion; Medical Care; Medications; Nutrition; Safety; Your Aging Body.

Write to the National Institute on Aging, Information Center, P.O. Box 8057, Gaithersburg, MD 20898-8057 for a complete list of their free publications.

The CONSUMER INFORMATION CENTER, P.O. Box 100, Pueblo, CO 81002 publishes a quarterly, "Consumer Information Catalog." This is a wonderful catalog that lists over 200 titles, either free or under $1.50, covering a variety of practical, useful subjects such as drugs and health aids, medical problems, mental health, and general health. Examples of some current titles include:

"Dizziness"	"The Menopause Time of Life"
"Facing Surgery"	"Do-It-Yourself Medical Testing"
"The Colon"	"Food and Drug Interactions"
"Gallstones"	"Some Things You Should
"Heart Attacks"	Know About Prescription Drugs"
"Osteoporosis"	

The FDA Consumer is a publication by the U.S. Food and Drug Administration. It provides information and reports on new medicines, their benefits and side effects, health advice of special concern to the elderly, and discussions of topics like sodium, osteoporosis, and generic drugs. *The FDA Consumer* is the official magazine of the FDA, which serves as the consumer protection agency responsible for food, drugs, medical devices, and other products used in daily life. A one-year subscription (10 issues) is $12. Write: FDA Consumer, Superintendent of Documents, Washington, D.C. 20402-9371.

ELDER-ED, P.O. Box 416, Kensington, MD 20795, has a free booklet entitled "Using Your Medicines Wisely: A Guide for the Elderly."

Write the AMERICAN COLLEGE OF SURGEONS, Office of Public Information, 55 East Erie Street, Chicago, IL 60611 for a free booklet on "When You Need An Operation." Or send for "Thinking of Having Surgery", Surgery HHS, Washington, D.C. 20201.

For free information on high blood pressure and diet write the HIGH BLOOD PRESSURE INFORMATION CENTER, 120/80, National Institutes of Health, Box AP, Bethesda, MD 20892.

CALLING THE SENIOR HELPLINE

Even with all the information available on aging, many older people, their caregivers, and families have trouble finding the right information when they need it most.

The national SENIOR HELPLINE was developed by the Gerontology Resource Center at Brigham Young University as a free service with answers on subjects ranging from family and finances to health and housing. By calling a toll-free number, seniors in all 50 states and Puerto Rico can hear short messages that are easily understood, interesting, and informative.

For example, a caller concerned about health problems can listen to messages on Alzheimer's Disease, alcoholism, bladder control, blood pressure, nutrition, and osteoporosis. There is also a free directory which, in addition to listing the message topics, includes names and addresses of foundations and professional organizations that can provide in-depth help on selected topics.

One of the benefits of the Helpline is the complete privacy in which a caller can listen to a message on a topic they may not wish to share with others. The toll-free number for the directory of messages and access codes is: (800) 328-7576. To obtain a written directory write: BYU Senior Helpline, F 274 HFAC, Brigham Young University, Provo, Utah 84602.

HEALTH NEWSLETTERS

Although there are several health newsletters available to the general public published by educational institutions, the *John Hopkins Medical Letter: Health After 50* is the first health newsletter specifically targeted for this age group. It is available from the Johns Hopkins Medical Institution, Dept. P, 550 N. Broadway, Suite 1100, Baltimore, MD 21205. The cost is $24 for 12 issues.

In addition, a growing number of companies and corporations are communicating health information to older workers and retirees through company newsletters and special mailings. The BANK OF AMERICA and LEVI STRAUSS are two examples of companies that provide their retirees with free newsletters and self-help books containing information on health promotion and maintenance. THE CENTER FOR CORPORATE HEALTH PROMOTION, one of the Travelers Companies, has developed a series of materials that address concerns of older adults. For information on these materials write: George J. Pfeiffer, Center for Corporate Health Promotion, Reston, VA.

FROM THE HEART

THE AMERICAN HEART ASSOCIATION publishes free reports and brochures covering all types of heart disease. They offer a variety of positive/preventative tips for maintaining a healthy cardiovascular system. For a list of publications write: American Heart Association, National Center, 7320 Greenvile Avenue, Dallas, TX 75231, or contact your local chapter of the American Heart Association.

NATIONAL ORGANIZATIONS AND PREVENTION PROGRAMS

Many national organizations provide free information on specific areas of health and disease prevention. Since many of these conditions begin to appear when we are older, we've included groups that offer materials on the more common health problems of mature adults.

THE AMERICAN RHEUMATISM ASSOCIATION offers information, brochures, and background publications on arthritis and other related conditions. Write: American Rheumatism Association, 17 Executive Park Drive, Suite 4809, Atlanta, GA 30329.

If you or a relative have arthritis and want more information, write to: THE ARTHRITIS FOUNDATION, P.O. Box 19000, Atlanta, GA 30326. The foundation has 70 chapters throughout the United States that offer courses and support resources designed to help arthritis patients and their families.

THE NATIONAL JEWISH CENTER FOR IMMUNOLOGY AND RE-SPIRATORY DISEASES will send you free brochures and publications by writing: Public Relations, National Jewish Center, 1400 Jackson Street, Denver, CO 80206.

BLUE SHIELD OF CALIFORNIA has a Senior Healthtrac program included with their Blue Shield Medicare Supplement plan. This is a computerized health management program with recommendations for staying healthy. For free information write: Mike Odom/Public Relations, Blue Shield of California, Two North Point, San Francisco, CA 94133 (Learn more about this program in Chapter 2).

THE NATIONAL OSTEOPOROSIS FOUNDATION, 1625 Eye Street, N.W., Suite 822, Washington, D.C. 20006, provides booklets and information regarding this disease, which is most prevalent in older women. In addition, PHYSICAL THERAPY SERVICES of Washington, D.C., Inc. has produced the *Osteoporosis Exercise Booklet* describing easy-to-do exercises designed to increase bone mass. Send $1.50 to Physical Therapy Services of Washington, D.C., Inc., 1145 19th St., N.W., Washington, D.C. 20036.

THE U.S. DEPARTMENT OF HEALTH AND HUMAN SERVICES administers a special funding program called the Hill-Burton Program, which requires hospitals and health facilities to provide services to people unable to pay. Those services are available to anyone residing in the facility's area. For information on the program, write your regional office of the Department of Health and Human Services or call the hot line toll free number: (800) 638-0742.

THE NATIONAL DIGESTIVE DISEASES EDUCATION AND IN-FORMATION CLEARINGHOUSE, Box NDDIC, Bethesda, MD 20892 offers free information on this subject.

Other national associations that provide free consumer health information include:

AMERICAN DIABETES ASSOCIATION, National Service Center, 1660 Duke Street, Alexandria, VA 22314, (800) 232-3472.

ALZHEIMER'S ASSOCIATION, 70 East Lake Street, Chicago, IL 6060l, (800) 621-0379.

NATIONAL KIDNEY FOUNDATION, 2 Park Avenue, New York, NY, 10003, (212) 889-2210.

NATIONAL MENTAL HEALTH ASSOCIATION, 1021 Prince Street, Alexandria, VA 22314, (703) 604-7722.

"HEALTH PEOPLE 2000"

This is a new federal program administered by the Department of Health and Human Services with the purpose of improving the health of all Americans by the year 2000. Its objectives are to reduce preventable death, disease, and disability, primarily by encouraging people to adopt healthy life-styles. The plan includes 30 objectives that are geared to the specific needs of older adults. Supporting these objectives, the AARP has launched a "Healthy Older Adults 2000" educational campaign with special focus on healthy life-styles. among Americans 50 years of age and older. The HHS overall plan will rely on industry, government, and local volunteers working together to achieve its goals. The AARP's focus is bringing the program to health and aging professionals and providing information directly to older consumers. For more information write: Health Advocacy Services, AARP, 1909 K St., N.W., Washington, D.C. 20049.

PLAN YOUR DAYS WITH THE
SENIOR WELLNESS CALENDAR

For the fifth year in a row, THE NATIONAL COUNCIL ON THE AGING has printed The Senior Wellness Calendar, featuring color photos of older Americans engaged in healthful activities. It also promotes monthly good health themes such as nutrition, walking for fitness, special health requirements for older women, and proper uses of medicines. The calendar costs $4 and can be obtained from The National Council on the Aging, Dept. 5087, Washington, D.C. 20061-50087.

HELP FOR OTHER HEALTH CONCERNS

Some health concerns affect older adults more than younger segments of the population. This often results from the natural effects of growing older. Although the process cannot always be stopped, there are preventive tests and positive measures that can greatly slow down their occurrence. Listed below are places and phone numbers where you can obtain additional information on preventative care for some of the more common health problems.

For most of us our eyesight has already begun to change and may continue to change throughout our later years. In addition to changes in vision, more than 90 percent of Americans over 65 develop cataracts—but they vary in seriousness, and only a small percentage require surgery. Recent research has shown that drugs, including simple aspirin, and certain vitamins may help prevent and significantly reduce a person's risk of developing cataracts. Some studies have even linked smoking and prolonged exposure to the sun to the risk of developing this condition. For free information send a self-addressed business-size envelope to the Inquiry Clerk in Department CT, the AMERICAN ACADEMY of OPHTHALMOLOGY, P.O. Box 7424, San Francisco, CA 94120.

THE VISION FOUNDATION, 2818 Mt. Auburn Street, Watertown, MA 02172 will send you a free "Vision Inventory List." THE NATIONAL SOCIETY TO PREVENT BLINDNESS, 500 East Remington Road, Schaumburg, IL 60173 has a free booklet called, *The Aging Eye: Facts on Eye Care for Older Persons.*

Another highly treatable problem that often does not show up until later in life is skin cancer. Since it sometimes take 20 years or more to develop following overexposure to the sun, skin cancer's incidence increases with age.

May is "National Skin Cancer & Detection Month." THE AMERICAN ACADEMY OF DERMATOLOGY can tell you what doctors in your area are giving free screenings. Call them at (708) 869-3954 or look for announcements in senior newspapers. Or check directly with the health facilities, clinics, and hospitals in your area for when they conduct low-cost or free exams.

In California, THE SKIN CANCER INSTITUTE (800-445-3926) offers free examinations for senior citizens 62 or older, or for anyone of any age with previous skin cancer. The CANCER DETECTION CENTER, a nonprofit corporation operating in Los Angeles since 1944, conducts periodic free skin cancer exams along with low-cost physical examinations for both men and women.

THE NATIONAL BREAST CANCER SCREENING CONSORTIUM offers a free informational brochure by sending a self-addressed stamped envelope to P.O. Box 4333, Grand Central Station, New York, NY 10163-4333. THE AMERICAN CANCER SOCIETY (800-227-2345) actively promotes nationwide low-cost mammogram programs during the year, especially in October during National Breast Cancer Awareness Month.

Private and public health facilities cooperate with these screening and information programs. THE NATIONAL ALLIANCE OF BREAST CANCER ORGANIZATIONS has over 220 member organizations around the country. They function as a resource network by sending out free pamphlets and articles and referring individuals to their members for consultation, screening, and information. If you have any questions write them at: National Alliance of Breast Cancer Organizations, 1180 Avenue of the Americas, 2nd Floor, New York, NY 10036.

Many men past the age of 40 develop prostate disorders, which in most cases are treatable with a simple outpatient procedure. In Los Angeles, THE BROTMAN MEDICAL CENTER (213-202-4766) offers free prostate screenings. Call the medical centers in your area to see if they offer similar screenings.

Another common concern among older adults is the flu. A yearly vaccine for seniors 55 and older is highly recommended, as well as a one-time dose of pneumonia vaccine. The idea that you can develop some kind of natural and lasting immunity to influenza is not true since flu viruses may change from year to year. The current vaccine has been proven to be very safe and effective about 80 percent of the time, greatly decreasing the risks of complications from flu.

Free and low-cost flu shots are provided by dozens of county health departments, health maintenance organizations, nursing homes, and community centers. They are given at local hospitals, senior centers, parks, banks, and other public sites. For example, FHP Health Care provides free shots at various FHP Centers.

THE NATIONAL COALITION FOR ADULT IMMUNIZATION (NCAI) has a public education program that begins during Adult Immunization Week in October of each year. Booklets and information sheets are available through the NCAI, National Foundation for Infectious Diseases, 4733 Bethesda Ave., Suite 750, Bethesda, MD 20814. Also THE NATIONAL INSTITUTE OF ALLERGY AND INFECTIOUS DISEASES, Box AP, Bldg., 31, Rm. 7A32, Bethesda, MD 20892 will send you a free booklet entitled *On Flu.*

Finally, a free 12-page pamphlet titled "Immunization of Adults: A Call to Action" and a "Lifetime Personal Immunization Record" are available from the CENTER FOR DISEASE CONTROL, Center For Prevention Services, Division of Immunization, Atlanta, GA 30333.

Dental problems and tooth loss do not have to be a serious problem for older people. In fact, losing teeth is not a normal part of aging. Over 60 percent of people 65 and older have their natural teeth. However, it is necessary to continue regular check-ups and treatment throughout your life. It has been proven that good oral health can affect and actually improve overall health. Unfortunately, Medicare does not pay for most dental care, and few older persons have separate dental insurance. This means the vast majority of dental services received are paid for out-of-pocket.

One way to reduce the high cost of dental care is through treatment at one of the 57 accredited dental schools in this country and Canada. Most of them provide patient care at 50 percent or more off most services. Many also provide special free services for the community-at-large, such as care to nursing home patients, oral cancer screenings at senior centers, and staff training to consumer groups. In addition, recent federal legislation has made the 15,000 nursing homes in this country receiving federal dollars directly responsible for the dental care needs of their residents.

There are over 200 dental hygiene programs across the country that provide special services for older persons. To find out about a program in your area contact your local dental society (listed in the phone book) or write one of the following:

AMERICAN ASSOCIATION OF DENTAL SCHOOLS
1625 Massachusetts Avenue, N.W.
Washington, D.C. 20036

AMERICAN DENTAL ASSOCIATION
211 East Chicago Avenue
Chicago, IL 60611

AMERICAN SOCIETY FOR GERIATRIC DENTISTRY
211 East Chicago Avenue, 16th Floor
Chicago, IL 60611

Several years ago, Ronald Reagan acknowledged that he wore a hearing aid. His revelation went a long way toward removing the stigma associated with these devices. More recently, senior citizen celebrities Like Richard Dysart and Eddie Albert have spoken out publicly about the benefits of hearing aids. LIke any health concern, hearing loss is most effectively treated if diagnosed early. The following are sources of free and low-cost hearing exams.

To find a otolaryngologist (ear, nose, and throat doctor), or an otologist (ear-only specialist), write to Physician's List, AMERICAN ACADEMY OF OTOLARYNGOLOGY, HEAD AND NECK SURGERY, One Prince St., Alexandria, VA 22314. Enclose a SASE to receive a free list of doctors in your area.

If you think you might have a hearing problem, you can contact SELF HELP FOR HARD OF HEARING PEOPLE (SHHH). They offer low-cost publications on dealing with hearing problems and a list of over 200 support groups around the country. Send a SASE to: SHHH, 7800 Wisconsin Ave., Bethesda, MD 20814.

THE BETTER HEARING INSTITUTE'S HEARING HELPLINE provides information on all kinds of hearing problems. Contact THE AMERICAN SPEECH-LANGUAGE-HEARING ASSOCIATION, 10801 Rockville Pike, Rockville, MD 20852, (800) 638-8255 for information on hearing and help in finding an audiologist (a professional trained to assess hearing loss)The toll-free number is (800) 327-9355..

THE COUNCIL FOR BETTER HEARING AND SPEECH, 5021-b Backlick Road, Annandale, VA 22003, (800) EAR-WELL will send you a free resource book.

BELTONE ELECTRONICS, one of the largest manufacturers of hearing aids, offers free hearing tests at their centers during Better Hearing Month (May). They will also send a free nonoperating model of their most popular canal hearing aid to show prospective users how tiny and light a hearing aid can be. To send for the model write: Dept. 14829, Beltone Electronics, 4201 West Victoria Street, Chicago, IL 60646.

The AARP publishes a report to help older people understand why hearing often declines with age and what products are on the market to help the problem. The report also offers tips on selecting the right equipment. For a free copy send a postcard to Product Report: Hearing Aids (D13766), AARP Fulfillment (EE118), 1909 K St. N.W., Washington, D.C. 20049.

Finally, there is a new telephone service called DIAL A HEARING SCREENING TEST (DAHST). The toll-free national number (800-222-3277) will direct you to a local number to take the test. When you call the test number, you receive complete instructions for taking the test, which consists of four soft tones for each ear.

In addition to general problems associated with hearing loss, there are about 6 million people who suffer from tinnitus, a ringing in the ears of bell-like sounds. The symptoms of tinnitus, which occurs more frequently in older persons, cause many people to suffer from sleeplessness, stress, and job-related difficulties. These symptoms are sometimes referred to as Meniere's disease when they include vertigo and dizziness, and can also be associated with hearing loss and fluctuation.

For information on tinnitus or a free copy of a brochure titled "Information About Tinnitus," write to: AMERICAN TINNITUS ASSOCIATION, P.O. Box 5, Portland, OR 97207. There is also a Meniere's Network, which publishes a booklet entitled, "An Introduction to Meniere's Disease." For a copy write: The EAR Foundation at Baptist Hospital, 2000 Church St., Box 111, Nashville, TN 37236 or call (800) 545-HEAR.

Many older people dismiss it, but feet and leg pains may be warning signs of more serious disorders and shouldn't be dismissed. They could be symptoms of a circulatory disorder called peripheral arterial disease, or P.A.D. There are many causes of P.A.D.—all either preventable or controllable. They are diabetes, high blood pressure, high cholesterol levels, and smoking. Smoking is number one. These can all cause restricted blood flow to the legs because of blockage in the arteries resulting in P.A.D. and possible further complications.

For information on P.A.D. write: THE CENTER FOR VASCULAR DISEASE, George Washington Medical University Center, 2150 Pennsylvania Ave., N.W., Washington, D.C. 20037 or THE AMERICAN DIABETES ASSOCIATION, INC., National Center, 1660 Duke St., Alexandria, VA 22314. Also the HOECHST-ROUSSEL PHARMACEUTICAL COMPANY, CME-MO, Dept. PAD, P.O. Box 830, Andover, NJ 078231 has produced a pamphlet called *Step Lively*, which they will send for free with a SASE.

As for our feet and toes, studies show that nearly 90 percent of Americans suffer at one time or another from foot ailments. These can result in headaches, fatigue, grouchiness, and lowered productivity. Some of the more common foot ailments include bunions, heel spurs, corns and calluses, fungus infections, and foot cramps. Check with local podiatry clinics, medical centers, and private podiatry groups for free or low-cost foot exams and an evaluation of what's ailing your feet. For example, in Los Angeles the CULVER CITY PODIATRY GROUP's advertisements include a coupon for a free foot exam worth $55.

WEAR A REAL LIFESAVER

In recent years several companies have come out with medical alert tags and identification cards which contain vital information for police, paramedics, and hospital staffs in case of a medical emergency. Although initially designed with children in mind, they have become very popular with older adults as well.

LIFESAVER CHARITIES OF CALIFORNIA produces a tear-resistant, washable tag that can be sewn into clothing or laced into shoes. The tag has space for name, address and phone number, phone numbers for friends or relatives, blood type, allergies, insurance company, and physician's number. The Lifesaver Tag is available free of charge by sending a SASE to: Lifesaver Charities, P.O. Box 2533, Garden Grove, CA 92640.

MEDICALERT is a nonprofit organization whose sole purpose is to notify emergency health care professionals to a person's special conditions. MedicAlert bracelets and necklaces alert attending persons to conditions such as asthma, heart problems, epilepsy, allergies, or diabetes. A lifetime membership in MedicAlert is $25 which includes a steel necklace or bracelet engraved with your personal identification number and a 24 hour call-collect telephone number tied into a data bank in California. As a backup you also get an identification card. Personal medical information is updated each year. To join, write MedicAlert Foundation International, Turlock, CA 95381-1009 or call (800) 432-5378.

For persons living alone, CARE ALERT emergency response service provides a small signal device worn by a person, which when pressed, signals the Emergency Center that a crisis is in progress. Paramedics are dispatched immediately, and neighbors and relatives are contacted. Care Alert also offers a free Medi-Guard bracelet or necklace and emergency card to anyone who signs up for the emergency response service. The response system operates automatically, 24 hours a day. For information call: (800) 593-0911.

WHITECROSS INTERNATIONAL CORP., 301 North Harrison Street, Ste. 440, Princeton, NJ 08540, (800) 874-6468, sells two laser-engraved BIOCARDs and attachments for $10

Micro-Med is a durable, laminated, wallet-sized card containing comprehensive medical information and a signature line authorizing medical personnel to begin emergency treatment immediately. The cost is $19. For information call (213) 851-3989.

DISCOUNTS ON DRUGS

In our chapter on associations, we mention several senior citizen clubs and groups that offer their members discounts on prescription medicines. Many of them offer mail-order services as well. In addition, LUCKY STORES, operating 100 pharmacies in California and Southern Nevada, have a "Lucky 60 Club" whereby anyone 60 or older can receive a 10 percent discount on prescription medications purchased at any Lucky Pharmacy. CVS PHARMACIES, with over 800 stores in 14 states covering the Northeast and California, also offer folks over 60 a 10 percent discount on prescriptions. (Customers in New Jersey must be 62 or older).

Ask at your local pharmacy whether they offer senior discounts for medicines and prescription drugs, either through their own club or membership in a senior organization.

CHAPTER 8

F.Y.I.: ASSOCIATIONS AND ORGANIZATIONS THAT WORK FOR MATURE ADULTS

There are more people in this country over the age of 55 than there are children in elementary and high school. Mature adults represent a major influence and power that affects nearly every area of American life. In addition to their growing numbers, they control most of this nation's disposable income. As a consequence this group has become a prime target of today's marketplace and a major concern and focus for our lawmakers and politicians.

A large number of national, state, and local organizations, some independent and some linked by vast networks of affiliates, have been created over the past few decades in the United States and Canada. These groups act as advocates and protectors of the rights of those 50 and over. Together, they represent millions of voices demanding action, attention, and respect. Not only do they provide important information and powerful lobbying services, but many offer special discounts and services for seniors that allow them to enjoy and accomplish many things in life that they would otherwise be unable to afford.

Organizations and associations that operate specifically to serve the needs of mature adults are listed below. By learning about these different groups you can choose which one(s) most closely match your interests and concerns as a mature adult. There is an enormous amount of information as well as services waiting to be discovered. There are also endless avenues available for working with these groups to improve the quality of life for yourself and other determined, dedicated seniors.

FEDERAL AGENCIES

Uncle Sam provides us with a wealth of information just for the asking. Below are government agencies that collect and distribute information to the public.

U.S. Department of Commerce
Bureau of the Census
Data User Services Division
Washington, D.C. 20233
(301) 763-4100
Census History Staff
(301) 763-7936

Within the Bureau of the Census is the Census History Staff. As an outgrowth of the collection of data from the census, the "Age Search Program" was begun. This program helps mature adults obtain personal historical information by requesting census records. These census records can help prove age and/or citizenship, and help to obtain a Birth Certificate, passport, or social security benefits.

U.S. Department of Health and Human Services
NATIONAL CENTER FOR HEALTH SERVICES RESEARCH AND HEALTH
Care Technology Assessment
Parklawn Building, Room 18-12
5600 Fishers Lane
Rockville, MD 20857
(301) 443-4100

This agency publishes reports on issues affecting the elderly, especially on the subject of Long Term Care. Contact them and request their list of free publications.

SOCIAL SECURITY ADMINISTRATION
6401 Security Blvd.
Baltimore, MD 21235
(301) 965-3120
(800) 2345-SSA (800-234-5772)
Local Social Security offices can help in finding out about senior programs, community groups, and activities in an area. The above

toll-free Social Security Administration telephone number operates from 7 A.M. to 7 P.M. throughout the country. Call during off-peak hours, such as 7 to 9 A.M. and 5 to 7 P.M. to receive free information on Social Security Programs, card name changes, earnings statements, Medicare, and Medicaid benefits.

U.S. Department of Health and Human Services
NATIONAL CENTER FOR HEALTH STATISTICS
3700 East-West Highway
Hyattsville, MD 20782
(301) 436-8509

This agency collects data regarding numerous health issues and produces reports for public use. Call them and request to be put on their mailing list. The free reports are published in pamphlets, which most often are summaries on issues of health. Any person on the mailing list is eligible for ordering the in-depth reports, usually 100 pages or more. Request the list of reports that focus particularly on "Health and the Aged" and order the ones that interest you.

NATIONAL INSTITUTE ON AGING
NIA Information Center
2209 Distribution Circle
Silver Springs, MD 20901
(301) 496-1752

The National Institute on Aging (NIA) offers free publications that can be ordered from the Public Information Office. Topics include clinical reports and summaries (i.e., Normal Human Aging, Special Reports on Aging), health education and disease prevention, research grants and training opportunities, diseases/disorders, health promotion, medical care, medications, nutrition, and safety.

U.S. Department of Labor
EMPLOYMENT & TRAINING ADMINISTRATION
DIVISION OF OLDER WORKERS PROGRAMS
200 Constitution Avenue, N.W.
Washington, D.C. 20210
(202) 535-0778

This is an especially helpful service if you are looking for employment or job training. Currently, the Division of Older Workers offers the following programs:

1. As a result of the Older American Act, the "Part-Time Employment Program" was created for people over age 55. It provides jobs working in community services run by government agencies or nonprofit organizations.

2. Under the Job Training Partnership Act, all ages are eligible for job training services, however 3 percent of those services (job training) and job placements must be for persons over the age of 55.

Another source to contact regarding employment at the local level is your State Office on Aging.

ADMINISTRATION ON AGING (AOA)
330 Independence Ave., S.W.
Washington, D.C. 20201
(202) 619-0724

This umbrella organization functions to oversee all the state Departments on Aging and the Areas Agencies on Aging offices around the United States. The focus of these organizations is to provide help to mature adults.

AREA AGENCY ON AGING (AAA)

There are 670 Area Agencies on Aging that assist mature Americans throughout the United States, assuring such needed services as delivery of hot meals, chore services, energy assistance, adult day care, and transportation assistance. AAA coordinates services for older adults in specific geographic areas. It is an excellent resource for learning about programs for 65+ adults within a specific locale. AAA's are found by checking in the "Blue Pages" of the telephone directory or contacting the State Office of Aging.

STATE AGENCIES

STATE OFFICES ON AGING/ STATE SENIOR DISCOUNT PRO-GRAMS: This public organization, also referred to as the "State Unit on Aging," serves as the focal point for all matters relating to the needs of mature persons within a given state. Each state has an Office on Aging as do the District of Columbia and the U.S. territories. You can find your state Office on Aging from one of the following:

- One of the state's Area Agencies on Aging.

- The Administration on Aging.

- The National Association of State Units on Aging.

- The Governor's Office.

Or contact the state office listed below. An example of some of the senior services and programs provided include: state senior discounts, senior passport programs, free hunting and fishing licenses, discounts on state park entrance fees and state camping facilities and Long-Term Aging Care, Senior Companion, Brown Bag, Health Care, Adult Day Health Care, Nutrition.

ALABAMA
Commission on Aging
State Capitol
Montgomery, AL 36130
(205) 261-5743

ALASKA
Older Alaskans Commission
C-Mail Station 0209
Juneau, AK 99811
(907) 465-3250

ARIZONA
Aging and Adult
Administration
1400 West Washington St.
Phoenix, AZ 85007
(602) 255-4446

ARKANSAS
Office of Aging and
Adult Services
Donaghey Building
7th and Main Streets
Little Rock, AR 72201
(501) 371-2441

CALIFORNIA
Department of Aging
1020 19th Street
Sacramento, CA 95814
(916) 322-5290

COLORADO
Aging and Adult
Service Division
Department of
Social Services
717 17th Street
Denver, CO 80218
(303) 294-5913

CONNECTICUT
Department of Aging
175 Main Street
Hartford, CT 06106
(203) 566-3238

DELAWARE
Division on Aging
Department of Health
and Social Services
1901 North Dupont Highway
New Castle, DE 19720
(302) 421-6791

DISTRICT OF COLUMBIA
Office of Aging
1424 K Street, N.W.
Washington, D.C. 20011
(202) 724-5626

FLORIDA
Program Office of Aging and
Adult Services
1317 Winewood Blvd.
Tallahassee, FL 32301
(904) 488-8922

GEORGIA
Office of Aging
878 Peachtree Street, N.E.
Atlanta, GA 30309
(404) 894-5333

HAWAII
Executive Office on Aging
Office of the Governor
335 Merchant Street
Honolulu, HI 96813
(808) 548-2593

IDAHO
Office on Aging
Statehouse Room 114
Boise, ID 83720
(208) 334-3833

ILLINOIS
Department on Aging
421 East Capitol Avenue
Springfield, IL 62701
(217) 785-2870

INDIANA
Department on Aging
and Community Services
251 North Illinois Street
Indianapolis, IN 46207
(317) 232-7006

IOWA
Department of Elder Affairs
914 Grand Avenue
Des Moines, IA 50319
(515) 281-5187

KANSAS
Department on Aging
610 West Tenth
Topeka, KS 66612
(913) 296-4986

KENTUCKY
Division for Aging Services
Department of Human
Resources
275 East Main Street
Frankfort, KY 40601
(502) 564-6930

LOUISIANA
Office of Elderly Affairs
P.O. Box 80374
Baton Rouge, LA 70898
(504) 925-1700

MAINE
Bureau of Maine's Elderly
State House, Station No. 11
Augusta, ME 04333
(207) 289-2561

MARYLAND
Office on Aging
301 W. Preston St.
Baltimore, MD 21201
(301) 225-1100

MASSACHUSETTS
Department of Elder Affairs
38 Chauncey St.
Boston, MA 02111
(617) 727-7750

MICHIGAN
Office of Services
to the Aging
P.O. Box 30026
Lansing, MI 48909
(517) 373-8230

MINNESOTA
Board on Aging
204 Metro Square Building
7th and Roberts Streets
St. Paul, MN 55101
(612) 296-2544

MISSISSIPPI
Council on Aging
301 West Pearl St.
Jackson, MS 39203
(601) 949-2070

MISSOURI
Division on Aging
Department of
Social Services
505 Missouri Blvd.
Jefferson City, MO 65102
(314) 751-3082

MONTANA
Community Services
Division
P.O. Box 4210
Helena, MT 59604
(406) 444-3865

NEBRASKA
Department on Aging
301 Centennial Mall-South
Lincoln, NE 68509
(402) 471-2306

NEVADA
Division on Aging
Department of
Human Resources
505 East King Street
Carson City, NV 89710
(702) 885-4210

NEW HAMPSHIRE
Council on Aging
105 London Road
Building No. 3
Concord, NH 03301
(603) 271-2751

NEW JERSEY
Division on Aging
Department of
Community Affairs
363 West State Street
Trenton, NJ 08625
(609) 292-4833

NEW MEXICO
State Agency On Aging
224 East Palace Avenue
Santa Fe, NM 87501
(505) 827-7640

NEW YORK
Office for the Aging
New York State Plaza
Agency Building No. 2
Albany, NY 12223
(518) 474-4425

NORTH CAROLINA
Division on Aging
1985 Umpstead Drive
Raleigh, NC 27603
(919) 733-3983

NORTH DAKOTA
Aging Services
Department of
Human Services
State Capitol
Bismarck, ND 58505
(701) 224-2577

OHIO
Department on Aging
50 West Broad Street-
9th Floor
Columbus, OH 42315
(614) 466-5500

OKLAHOMA
Special Unit on Aging De-
partment of Human Services
P.O. Box 25352
Oklahoma City, OK 73125
(405) 521-2281

OREGON
Senior Services Division
313 Public Service Building
Salem, OR 97310
(503) 378-4728

PENNSYLVANIA
Department of Aging
231 State Street
Harrisburg, PA 17101
(717) 783-1550

PUERTO RICO
Gericulture Commission
Department of
Social Services
P.O. Box 11398
Santurce, PR 00910
(809) 721-4010

RHODE ISLAND
Department of
Elderly Affairs
79 Washington Street
Providence, RI 02903
(401) 277-2858

SOUTH CAROLINA
Commission on Aging
915 Main Street
Columbia, SC 29201
(803) 758-2576

SOUTH DAKOTA
Office of Adult
Services and Aging
700 North Illinois Street
Pierre, SD 57501
(605) 773-3656

TENNESSEE
Commission on Aging
535 Church Street
Nashville, TN 37219
(615) 741-2056

TEXAS
Department on Aging
1949 IH-35 South
P.O. Box 12786
Capitol Station
Austin, TX 78741
(512) 444-2727

UTAH
Division of Aging and
Adult Services
Department of
Social Services
150 West North Temple
Salt Lake City, UT 84145
(801) 533-6422

VERMONT
Office on Aging
103 South Main Street
Waterbury, VT 05676
(802) 241-2400

VIRGIN ISLANDS
Commission on Aging
6F Havensight Mall
Charlotte Amalie
St. Thomas, VI 00801
(809) 774-5884

VIRGINIA
Department on Aging
18th Floor, 101
North 14th Street
Richmond, VA 23219
(804) 225-2271

WASHINGTON
Aging and Adult Services
Department of Social
and Health Services
OB-43G
Olympia, WA 98504
(206) 753-2502

WEST VIRGINIA
Commission on Aging
Holly Grove - State Capitol
Charleston, WV 25305
(304) 348-3317

WISCONSIN
Bureau of Aging
Division of Community
Services
One West Wilson Street
Madison, WI 53702
(608) 266-2536

WYOMING
Commission on Aging
Hathaway Building-Room 139
Cheyenne, WY 82002
(307) 777-7986

MORE PUBLIC AGENCIES

ACTION
1100 Vermont Ave., N.W.
Washington, D.C. 20525
(800) 424-8867

ACTION'S mission is to promote the spirit and practice of volunteering. Since 1964, this mission has been carried out by the more than half a million volunteers from all walks of life. ACTION programs include: Foster Grandparent Program (FGP), the Retired Volunteer Program (RSVP), the Senior Companion Program (SCP), Volunteers In Service To America (VISTA), the Student Community Service Program, and the ACTION Drug Alliance. The agency also provides grants, technical assistance, and a vast knowledge of volunteer resources, initiatives, and programs. The majority of volunteers in ACTION programs are older men and women, thousands of whom help young people who are at risk of dropping out of school, using drugs, or being physically abused or neglected. Through ACTION, older Americans show what tremendous contributions they can make to society. Volunteering through ACTION is a great way to commit your talents and skills to your country. As President Bush has stated, "From now on in America, any definition of a successful life must include service to others."

U.S. DEPARTMENT OF HEALTH AND HUMAN SERVICES
HEALTH CARE FINANCING ADMINISTRATION (HCFA)
(202) 296-2920; (202) 243-0312

HFMA is responsible for funding and administering the Medicare program. It also assists in the fulfilling of this responsibility for the various Medicaid programs. The agency is an excellent resource for information about health care expenses, use of medical services and insurance coverage for those 65 and older.

SERVICE CORPS OF RETIRED EXECUTIVES (SCORE)
Small Business Administration
1129 20th St., N.W.
Washington, D.C. 20036
(202) 653-6279

SCORE utilizes retired and semi-retired businessmen to counsel new and existing small businesses.

U.S. HOUSE SELECT COMMITTEE ON AGING
300 New Jersey Ave., S.E.
Room 712 Annex #1
Washington, D.C. 20515
(202) 226-3375

U.S. SENATE SPECIAL COMMITTEE ON AGING
Dirksen Office Building
Washington, D.C. 20510
(202) 224-5364

Both the House Select Committee on Aging and its counterpart in the Senate are great places to find out about existing, pending, or anticipated legislation involving older adults.

PRIVATE ORGANIZATIONS

American Association of Retired Persons

AMERICAN ASSOCIATION OF RETIRED PERSONS
Office of Communications
1909 K Street, N.W.
Washington, D.C. 20049
(202) 728-4300

AARP—the American Association of Retired Persons—is a nonprofit, nonpartisan organization dedicated to helping older Americans achieve lives of independence, dignity and purpose.

Founded in 1958, AARP is the nation's oldest and largest organization of older Americans, with a membership of more than 32 million. Membership is open to anyone age 50 or older, whether working or retired. AARP's motto is to "serve, not to be served."

Membership dues (including spouse) are $5 for one year, $12.50 for three years and $35 for 10 years. AARP members receive *Modern Maturity* magazine bimonthly and *AARP News Bulletin* 11 times per year. *Modern Maturity* has the second largest circulation of any U.S. magazine. The Association also distributes a wide range of specialized publications, many of which are available free of charge.

The Retired Teachers Division is open to former members of the National Retired Teachers Association and to soon-to-retire teachers, administrators, and other education professionals. Members receive NRTA News Bulletin and NRTA edition of Modern *Maturity magazine.*

AARP Priorities include four major areas that affect the quality of life that the AARP has targeted for a significant portion of its resources. These issue "initiatives" include: Health Care Campaign, Women's Initiative, Worker Equity, and Minority Affairs Initiative. AARP represents a diverse population that includes workers and retirees, women re-entering the workforce, frail women over 80 living alone, people with comfortable standards of living, and those who struggle daily. A major AARP commitment is the development of legislative policy recommendations serving such a diverse group of older Americans.

AARP Member Services: Purchase Privilege Program - Provides members with discounts at major car rental companies, motel and hotel chains, recreational and tourist facilities.

Pharmacy Service - Provides prescription medicines and other health care items to members by mail or direct purchase.

Travel Service - A wide variety of escorted or independent travel opportunities, i.e., tours, cruises, special-event programs and hosted living abroad programs, designed for AARP mature travelers.

AARP Motoring Service - Includes a customized plan provided by AMOCO Motor Club. Members of the AARP Motoring Plan receive 20 road service benefits.

Group Health Insurance - Underwritten for AARP members by the Prudential Insurance Company.

Auto/Homeowners Insurance - Offered by The Hartford Insurance Group to Association members.

Mobile Home Insurance - Insurance for mobile home owners is provided by the Foremost Insurance Group.

Educational Resources. AARP produces audiovisual program kits on issues ranging from health and nutrition, housing, and retirement planning to consumer protection and crime prevention. The kits are loaned free of charge to nonprofit organizations providing services to older people and members of the aging network.

The organization also publishes a continuing series of books of special usefulness and importance to middle-aged and older readers. Subjects include: money management, retirement planning, insurance decisions, foot care, crime prevention, widowhood, funeral planning, and housing alternatives.

AARP publications include more than 140 titles available free of charge upon request. These authoritative materials cover a variety of topics including health, consumer affairs, crime prevention, retirement planning, lifetime learning, and driver re-education. Information ranges from practical advice to "how-to" guides, demographics to resource publications. For a complete list of publications write: AARP Fulfillments, EE0073, 1909 K St., N.W., Washington, D.C. 20049.

Community Services. More than 400,00 AARP volunteers are involved in community service programs nationwide that reinforce self-worth and self-reliance among older people. Through these programs, older Americans are given the opportunity to share their wisdom, experience, and abilities with those of all ages in need.

Some other beneficial programs administered by the AARP and its more than 3,700 local chapters and 2,500 Retired Teacher Association units throughout the United States include:

Consumer Affairs Program; Criminal Justice Service; 55 Alive/Mature Driving; Health Advocacy Services; Housing Program; Institute of Lifetime Learning; Intergenerational Program; International Activities; Interreligious Liaison; Legal Counsel for the Elderly; National Gerontology Resource Center; National Retired Teachers Association Activities; Senior Community Service Employment Program; Tax Aide Program; Widowed Persons Service.

Sears Mature Outlook

Sears Mature Outlook
6001 N. Clark St.
Chicago, IL 60660-9977
1-800-336-6330.

Sponsored by Sears, the country's largest retailer, this club specializes in discounts, some of them substantial, on products and services in its stores, plus many other benefits for folks over 50. The annual fee is $9.95, which includes your spouse.
   Some of their services and benefits include:

Mature Outlook magazine, a readable, artfully designed magazine with articles and columns full of practical information aimed towards mature adults.

Mature Outlook Newsletter, also a source of useful facts and tips.

$100 in "Sears Money" that can be used like cash on any merchandise or Sears services. These certificates are unrestricted and can be used for purchases in any store or Sears catalog. "Bonus Club" merchandise certificates from Sears are issued for accumulated purchases to customers using Sears Charge accounts.

Automotive service: a coupon book redeemable at Sears Automotive Centers for discounts on various maintenance jobs.

"Travel Alert" with savings up to 35 percent to 50 percent for domestic and international tours, cruises, and last-minute bookings at even bigger savings.

Discounts of 20 percent off the room rates and 10 percent off meals at participating Holiday Inns and Crowne Plaza Hotels. Also discounts on car rentals from Budget/Sears, Hertz, Avis, and National.

Mail-order pharmacy discounts.

10 percent off the membership charge for the Allstate Motor Club.

20 precent discount on eyewear products at participating Sears Optical Departments. Plus "Vision One" membership for up to 50

percent on glasses, contacts, fashion frames, and eyecare services.

Savings on service fees on Citicorp Traveler's Checks.

$5,000 Travel Accident Insurance for members and $5,000 for their spouse.

Other Private Organizations

ADVOCATES SENIOR ALERT PROCESS
1334 G Street N.W.
Washington, D.C. 20005
(202) 737-6340

 Advocates Senior Alert Process—(A.S.A.P.) is a cooperative project of national senior organizations that are looking for volunteers who can give of their time. This group has won legislative battles by having concerned citizens write letters, make phone calls, and meet with representatives and senators working towards achieving affordable, quality health care for all Americans. Among their accomplishments has been the blocking of proposals to cut Social Security COLA's (cost-of-living-adjustments) in each of the past several years. Volunteer workers receive free information and booklets including: "Advocacy Tips," "A.S.A.P. Update," special reports and action alerts.

AMERICAN SENIOR CITIZEN ASSOCIATION (ASCA)
P. O. Box 41
Fayetteville, NC 20302
(919) 323-3641

The purpose of this organization is to promote the physical, mental, emotional, and economic well-being of senior citizens. Comprising 35,000 seniors, this group believes that senior citizens have the right to live with competence, security, and dignity. The ASCA promotes activities that encourage seniors to be active participants in the community.

ASSOCIATION OF INFORMED SENIOR CITIZENS
460 Spring Park Place, Suite 100
Herndon, VA 22070
(703) 437-7600

This association has served as a consumer interest group since 1981. There are currently 50,000 members made up of citizens 55 and older. They provide information and publish materials on services, discounts, and government-funded programs for senior citizens. Their publications include: "The AISC Reporter," " Guide Book on Federal Programs for the Elderly," "What You Should Know About Disability Benefits," and "What Your Doctor Should Know About Disability Benefits."

SENIOR CITIZENS LAW CENTER
1052 W. Sixth Street, Suite 700
Los Angeles, CA 90017
(213) 482-3550

This is a legal services support center specializing in the legal problems of the elderly. It acts as an advocate on behalf of elderly and poor clients in legislative and administrative affairs. Contact them for copies of handbooks, testimonies and guides.

AMERICAN SOCIETY ON AGING
833 Market Street, Suite 512
San Francisco, CA 94103
(415) 543-2617

Members include senior citizens, students, business persons, educators, researchers, administrators, health care and social service professionals who work to enhance the well being of older individuals and create unity among those working with and for the elderly. It focuses on the interests and needs of older people world-wide, particularly in the Third World. Besides offering continuing education programs on age-related issues, The American Society on Aging generates two important publications: *Generations*, a journal that provides practical current information in the field of aging, with emphasis on medical and social practice, research, and policy; and *The Aging Connection*, a bimonthly newspaper that covers critical events and issues in the field of aging.

NATIONAL INTERFAITH COALITION ON AGING
298 South Hull Street
Athens, GA 30603
(404) 353-1331

This group promotes and provides resources for ministries with older adults. NICA works with more than 25 Protestant, Jewish, Catholic, and Orthodox organizations to provide training and develop resources through local congregations and religious organizations. This group approaches senior issues by representing the spiritual concerns of older Americans in public and private forums. Membership is $35 a year.

CATHOLIC GOLDEN AGE
P.O. Box 3658
Scranton, PA 18505-0658
(800) 982-4367 (PA)
(800) 233-4697 (Rest of the U.S.)

A nonprofit association of senior citizens founded in 1975, Catholic Golden Age provides spiritual benefits as well as material benefits and discounts to men and women age 50 and over. Currently Catholic Golden Age has over 400,000 members. CGA member benefits, services, and privileges include:

- Spiritual benefits - The CGA Annual Eucharistic Liturgy, Million Candles Observance.

- CGA local chapter activities.

- *CGA World*, a bimonthly magazine that offers editorial on the social, physical, economic, intellectual and spiritual needs of older adults.

- Eyeglass discounts.

- Pharmacy services and discounts up to 50 percent on prescriptions and vitamins.

- CGA MasterCard/Visa - No annual fee the first year.

- Film processing discounts.

- Interstate moving discount from North American Van Lines, Inc.

- Car rental discount on Alamo, Avis, Dollar, Hertz, National, and Thrifty.

- Used car discount - Save $200 on Avis used cars.

- CGA motoring plan.
- Vacation and special attraction discounts.
- CGA group travel benefits.
- Gray Line Tours - Save 20 percent.
- Hotel/motel discounts of 10 to 50 percent off room rates at more than a dozen national hotel/motel chains.
- CGA group insurance plans.

JEWISH ASSOCIATION FOR SERVICES FOR THE AGED
40 W. 68th St.
New York, NY 10023
(212) 724-3200

Established on the East Coast in 1968, this social welfare organization provides the services necessary to enable older adults to remain in the community. There are over 60,000 members, served in New York City and Nassau and Suffolk counties. Services include: information and referral to appropriate health, welfare, educational, social, recreational, and vacation services, government benefits and entitlements; personal counseling; financial assistance; health and medical service counseling; counseling on housing and long-term care; homemaker service; group educational and recreational activities; hot lunch programs; referral to summer camps; legal services; protective services; reaching out to the isolated; programs for the independent senior clubs.

GRAY PANTHERS
1424 16th Street, N.W., Suite 602
Washington, D.C. 20036
(202) 387-3111

The Gray Panthers was founded in 1970 by social activist Maggie Kuhn and five friends. Today there are more than 70,000 members in this grassroots organization comprising young, old, and middle-aged citizens actively speaking up for older Americans. Over the years, Gray Panthers have lead the fight against forced retirement at age 65, exposed shocking nursing home abuses leading to convictions and tough new laws, and beat President Reagan's plans to increase military spending and ax programs such as Medicare and Medicaid. They support a number of social causes that oppose ageism and lobby in favor of extension of senior citizen rights and entitlements, promote intergenerational relationships, health care consumerism, Social Security, housing, nursing homes, and Medicare.

NATIONAL COUNCIL OF SENIOR CITIZENS
925 15th Street NW
Washington, D.C. 20077-2028
(202) 347-8800

A voice for older Americans, NCSC is an advocacy organization dedicated to the belief that America's elderly are worthy of the best that this nation can give. Founded in 1961, NCSC lobbies on the local, state, and national level for legislation benefiting older Americans. With about 4.5 million members in over 5,000 NCSC clubs, it has carried on many successful campaigns including increased Social Security benefits, creation of senior centers and nutrition sites, community employment projects, low-income senior housing and many other social services. Membership also includes: a local club network with social events and activities, discount prescription drug service by mail, Medicare supplemental health insurance, hospital income insurance for people under 65, travel and car rental discounts, and *Senior Citizen News,* an informative publication. Yearly dues are $8.

NATIONAL ASSOCIATION OF RETIRED FEDERAL EMPLOYEES
(NAFRE)
1533 New Hampshire Ave., NW
Washington, D.C. 20036
(202) 234-0832

This is an association of federal retirees and their families. They represent an aggressive lobbying force on Capitol Hill whose purpose is to protect retirement benefits. Membership includes an annual subscription to *Retirement Life* magazine, and membership in a local chapter. Other NAFRE benefits include:

Discounts on Avis and Hertz car rentals; Travel discounts; Up to 50 percent savings on worldwide cruises; NARFE VISA with no annual fee for six months; Vision care program with free sight evaluations and discounts on eyewear; 50 percent off rooms at 1500 Quest International hotels; United Airlines' Silver Wings Plus Travel Club membership for those over 60, plus tours, hotel, car-rental savings, and airline discounts; long-term care insurance plan. Membership is $16 a year.

ASSOCIATION OF RETIRED AMERICANS
P.O. Box 4398
Scottsdale, AZ 85261-9896

This is a nonprofit organization serving the needs of senior men and women. They offer a free Medicare Supplement Comparison Chart Analysis as part of their program to keep senior citizens informed about health and welfare rights and benefits.

NATIONAL ASSOCIATION FOR RETIRED CREDIT UNION PEOPLE (NARCUP)
P.O. Box 391
Madison, WI 53701

NARCUP's membership is open to retirees who are or were credit union members (and their spouses), or persons who are credit union members and are at least age 50. Their services and benefits help older adults plan for retirement and aid them in managing their resources effectively following retirement.

Membership includes a subscription to *Prime Times* magazine, retirement and management information booklets and seminars, consumer information, a choice of supplemental health insurance plans and a variety of travel services and travel discounts. NARCUP also offers discounts on prescription/pharmacy services by mail and a discount eyewear program. Membership is $12 for the first year and $7 for yearly renewals.

OLDER WOMEN'S LEAGUE
730 Eleventh Street NW, Suite 300
Washington, D.C. 2000l
(202) 783-6686

In this country, the problems of aging are largely women's problems.

- More than 70 percent of the nearly 4 million persons over 65 living in poverty are women.

- Fewer than 20 percent of older women currently receive any pension income.

- Most women over 65 depend on Social Security as their only significant income.

- Millions of mid-life women have no health insurance.

The Older Women's League works to change these facts. It is the first grassroots membership organization to focus exclusively on women as they age. OWL works to provide mutual support for its members, helps them achieve economic and social equity, and works to improve the image and status of older women. It provides educational materials, training for citizen advocates, and informational publications dealing with the important issues facing women as they grow older. Members are eligible for supplemental insurance plans, receive the *OWL Observer* newspaper, and receive discounts on all OWL publications. Membership is $10 yearly.

AMERICAN LEGION
1608 K St., N.W.
Washington, D.C. 20006
(202) 861-2711

The American Legion is the nation's largest veterans, organization. While it isn't made up solely of those 50+, it does include a large group of older veterans. *American Legion Magazine*, for example, has a circulation of more than 2.5 million. Its average reader is 60 years old. The Legion's most visible activity is its work on behalf of veterans, their survivors, and dependents. In addition, a large portion of the Legion's American resources are channeled into education programs and citizenship activities for youth. Each year more than 200 American Legion community service projects costing more than $5 million in aid touch the lives of millions of Americans.

Note: Service organizations such as the Rotary, Lions, Kiwanis, and Elks also have large age 50+ constituencies. These groups also have both local and regional clubs.

NATIONAL CAUCUS AND CENTER ON THE BLACK AGED
1424 K St., N.W., Suite 500
Washington, D.C. 20005
(202) 637- 8400

This organization seeks to improve living conditions for low-income elderly Black Americans. They advocate changes in federal and state laws by improving the economic, health, and social status of low-income senior citizens. They also promote community awareness of problems and issues affecting this group. It operates an employment program involving 2,000 older persons in 14 states and sponsors, owns, and manages rental housing for the elderly.

NATIONAL HISPANIC COUNCIL ON AGING
2713 Ontario Road, N.W.
Washington, D.C.
(202) 265-1288

Members of this organization work for the well-being of the Hispanic elderly through research, policy analysis, and projects, and provide a network for organizations and community groups interested in the Hispanic elderly.

NATIONAL ASSOCIATION OF HISPANIC ELDERLY
The Association Nacional Pro Personas Mayores
2727 West Sixth St. Suite 270
Los Angeles, CA 90057
(213) 487-1922

This organization focuses on helping rural elderly in southern Texas and northern California to gain access to supportive services offered under the Older Americans Act. Trained volunteers help the elderly obtain needed assistance and local services.

NATIONAL INDIAN COUNCIL ON AGING
P.O. Box 2088
Albuquerque, NM 87103

This organization seeks to bring about improved, comprehensive services to the Indian and Alaskan native elderly. It acts as a focal point
for the articulation of the needs of the Indian elderly, disseminate
information on Indian aging programs, provide technical assistance and
training opportunities to tribal organizations, and conduct research on
the needs of Indian elderly.

NATIONAL PACIFIC/ASIAN RESOURCE CENTER
2033 6th Avenue, Suite 410
Seattle, WA 98121
(206) 448-0313

This group's goals are to ensure and improve the delivery of health and
social services to elderly Pacific/Asians and increase the capabilities of
community-based services to the elderly. They also produce several
informative publications and national community service directory.

NATIONAL COMMITTEE TO PRESERVE SOCIAL SECURITY
AND MEDICARE (NCPSSM)
2000 K St., N.W., Suite 800
Washington, D.C. 20006
(202) 822-9459

The NCPSSM is a highly vocal organization and one of the largest
lobbying groups in America dealing with Social Security, Medicare, and
other senior issues on Capitol Hill.

NATIONAL ALLIANCE OF SENIOR CITIZENS (NASC)
2525 Wilson Blvd.
Arlington, VA 22201
(703) 528-4380

This national lobbying organization is targeted to a politically conserva-
tive audience. There are more than 2 million members working to
promote the advancement of senior Americans through sound fiscal
policy. Their purpose is to inform the American public of the needs of
senior citizens and of the programs and policies being carried out by
the government and other groups. Members' benefits include life insurance plan, VISA card with no fee for six months, newsletters, discounts

on lodging, car rentals, moving expenses, and a motoring club. Dues are $10 a year ($15 for a couple).

THE RETIRED OFFICERS ASSOCIATION
201 N. Washington St.
Alexandria, VA 22314-2529
(703) 549-2311

This association is an independent nonprofit organization dedicated to maintaining a strong national defense and preserving the entitlements and benefits of uniformed services personnel, their families, and survivors. TROA, with a membership of 365,000, is the largest military officers' association in the country. Members receive *The Retired Officers Magazine*, containing reports on Congress and matters of special interest. Other benefits include counseling in employment assistance, personal affairs, dependent scholarship loans/grants, survivor assistance, and retirement information. There are also discounts on car rentals, a discount travel program, health screenings, sports holidays, a mail-order prescription program, group health and life insurance plans, financial services, and an extended car warranty program. Yearly membership fees are $16.

CANADIAN ASSOCIATION OF RETIRED PERSONS (C.A.R.P.)
27 Queen Street East, Suite 304
Toronto, Ontario M5C 2M6
Canada
(800) 387-2092/(416) 363-8748

This organization is a national nonprofit, nonpolitical association of Canadians over 50 established to promote the interests of mature Canadians. Membership is $10 a year (including spouse). This group is the Canadian counterpart to the AARP, and in just five years has grown to an enrollment of 52,000 members. Benefits include "C.A.R.P. News" newsletter, discounts on health care, home and car insurance, car rentals, hotels, theaters, and travel.

CHAPTER 9

ADDITIONAL SUGGESTED READING

Throughout this book we have made reference to numerous booklets, newsletters, and periodicals that address the issues and concerns of mature Americans. We believe the more information and knowledge people have about a subject, the better equipped they are to make responsible and beneficial decisions leading to a higher quality of life. Of course, the decisions we make are not always the right ones, but the more information we have regarding the topics covered in this book, the better are our chances of making the correct decisions.

We encourage all of our readers who are faced with making important decisions during these years to explore every avenue and possibility that will help make those decisions as satisfying and fruitful as possible. Whether you plan to travel, look for retirement investments, go back to school, seek to improve your health, help others with their lives, etc., there are many considerations you will need to take into account before acting upon a decision.

In addition, the pleasure that comes from reading and learning is a gift we can enjoy throughout our entire lives. Reading keeps us current and informed on the latest developments concerning us as well as in the world around us. As mature adults, we can ill afford, to sit on our laurels and say, "Let the younger generations take it from here." The ones who are going to make life better for all mature adults are mature adults themselves. That is why the organizations in this book are among the most influential and powerful in the nation. So after finishing this book, read on and on and on. . . .You won't regret it.

MAGAZINES FOR THE MATURE MARKET

AGING
Human Development Services
Department of Health and Human Services
200 Independence Ave., SW
Washington, D.C. 20201

GENERATIONS
American Society on Aging
833 Market St., Suite 512
San Francisco, CA 94103

This excellent quarterly journal provides practical, current information in the field of aging, with emphasis on medical and social practice, research, and policy.

GOLDEN YEARS
233 E. New Haven Ave.
P.O. Box 537
Melbourne, FL 32902-0537
(407) 725-4888

A general interest magazine with features on travel, health, real estate, money matters, current events, family concerns, etc.

GRANDPARENTS TODAY
475 Park Avenue
New York, NY 10016
(212) 545-5353

LEAR'S
505 Park Avenue
New York, NY 10022

Targeted towards the sophisticated, educated, and active "woman who wasn't born yesterday", this up-scale monthly magazine covers a variety of topics including fashion, business, current books, health, and relationships.

LONGEVITY
1965 Broadway
New York, NY 10023-5965
(212) 496-6100

McCALLS SILVER EDITION
110 Fifth Avenue
New York, NY 10011
(212) 463-1000

This is an insert aimed towards mature adults published by *McCalls* magazine six times a year.

MATURE OUTLOOK
One North Arlington
1500 W. Shure Dr.
Arlington Heights, IL 60004
(800) 336-6330

This general-interest magazine is available with membership in Sear's Mature Outlook club. Includes features on travel, gardening, food, health, money, sports, etc., and promotes the benefits and savings available through club membership.

MERIDIAN
Troika Publishing Inc.
Box 13337
Kanata, ON K2K 1X5
Canada

This is a magazine covering the interests of Canadians over 55. Free subscriptions are offered to Canadians requesting it.

MODERN MATURITY
3200 E. Carson St.
Lakewood, CA 90712
(213) 496-2277

This is the official publication for the AARP. A subscription to the monthly magazine is included with membership in AARP. This consumer oriented publication covers a wide range of topics of interest to mature adults, including reports on the latest developments in AARP lobbying campaigns, current AARP publications, club services and benefits.

NEW CHOICES: FOR THE BEST YEARS
28 W. 23rd St.
New York, NY 10010
(212) 366-8800 (800) 347-6969 (magazine subscription)

New Choices is another general-interest monthly publication aimed at the mature adult market. It is published by *Reader's Digest*, and contains lots of articles of special interest to seniors plus practical and useful information.

New Choices also publishes a very good series of booklets entitled: "50 Plus Pre-Retirement Services". Some of the topics covered in the series include: health, leisure, retirement, single living, the law, housing, money, and Social Security benefits. Prices for booklets range from $3.50-$4 plus postage and can be ordered through New Choices, 50 Plus Guidebooks, P.O. Box 1945, Marion, Ohio 43305-1945.

PRIME TIMES
5910 Mineral Point Road
P.O. Box 391
Madison, WI 53701

This quarterly magazine is published for the members of the National Association of Retired Credit Union People. Subscriptions are also available to nonmembers. Its articles keep readers informed of new services, consumer issues, and relevant topics of interest.

RETIRED OFFICER MAGAZINE
201 North Washington St.
Alexandria, VA 22314-2529
(703) 549-2311

This publication, with a circulation of 365,000, is edited for the retired military community. It is the official publication of the Retired Officers Association. Its columns keep readers up to date with news from Capitol Hill and the Pentagon, as well as items of personal interest.

RETIREMENT LIFE
1533 New Hampshire Ave., N.W.
Washington, D.C. 20036

Retirement Life is the official magazine of the National Association of Retired Federal Employees. Published monthly, it informs the 495,000 members of the NARFE of important lobbying developments and legislative changes affecting the rights of older adults. Topics include Social Security, Medicare/Medicaid, supplemental insurance, elder abuse, COLAs, taxes, privacy rights.

SOLUTIONS FOR BETTER HEALTH
Haymarket Group
45 West 34th Street, #500
New York, NY 10001
(212) 239-0855

NEWSLETTERS

There are many newsletters that address areas of interest to mature adults, including retirement, travel, political issues, health and fitness, sports, etc. Some are targeted, specifically to those 50 and over, and others include special reports or new developments relating to this age group. Nearly every national agency, society, and association publishes a newsletter informing its membership of activities, events, etc., pertaining to the interests and objectives of the organization.

The following are a few examples of newsletter, that offer useful and interesting information:

THE MATURE TRAVELER
GEM Publishing
P.O. Box 50820
Reno, NV 89513
(702) 786-7419

THE RETIREMENT LETTER
Peter A. Dickinson, Editor
44 Wildwood Dr.
Prescott, AZ 86301

TRAVEL SMART (includes special items for seniors)
40 Beechdale Rd.
Dobbs Ferry, NY 10522

VITAL CONNECTIONS
Foundation for Grandparenting
P.O. Box 31
Lake Placid, NY 12946

MULTIPLE PUBLISHERS

Senior Publishers Group is made up of newspapers and magazines written, edited, and published for active, older adults. They represent 98 newspapers and magazines throughout the United States and Canada. To locate a senior newspaper or publication in your area write: SENIOR PUBLISHERS GROUP, 1326 Garnet Avenue, San Diego, CA 92109.

The AARP publishes many books with information on a variety of subjects of interest to mature adults. For a catalog of their publications write: AARP BOOKS, Scott, Foresman and Company, 1865 Miner Street, Des Plaines, IL 60016.

For a complete list of AARP publications including dozens of free booklets, audio-visual programs, posters, periodicals, newsletters, books, and legal counsel guides and handbooks, write for "AARP Publications & A/V Program: The Complete Collection", AARP, American Association of Retired Persons, 1901 K Street NW, Washington, D.C. 20049.

Senior Spectrum Newspapers publishes 19 senior newspapers serving communities in Northern and Central California and Northern Nevada. To find out about a newspaper in your area write: Senior Spectrum Newspapers, 9261 Folsom Blvd., Suite 401, Sacramento, CA, (916) 364-5454.

Pilot Books publishes several paperback directories listing travel discounts for mature adults. For a copy of their catalog write: Pilot Books 103 Cooper Street, Babylon, NY 11702.

BOOKS

As you can imagine, there are dozens of books covering dozens of subjects of interest to adults over 50. More than any other age group, mature adults are interested in ways to improve their health, maintain (or build) their wealth, and enjoy their "golden years" to the maximum. And that includes reading and learning from as many sources as are available. The following is a sampling of useful and informative books that represent some of the most popular areas of interest:

HEALTH

American Heart Association Cookbook. The American Heart Association. New York: Ballantine Books, $10.95.

Aquacises: Restoring and Maintaining Mobility with Water Exercises. Miriam Study Giles. Lexington, Mass.: Mills & Sanderson, $9.95.

At-A-Glance Nutrition Counter. Patricia Hausman. New York: Ballantine Books, $2.95.

Columbia Encyclopedia of Nutrition, compiled and edited by Myron Winick, M.D., and the Institute of Human Nutrition, Columbia University College of Physicians and Surgeons. G.P. Putnam's Sons, New York: $19.95.

The Complete Manual of Fitness and Well Being. Dr. Robert Arnot, Special Adviser. New York: Viking Penguin, $25.00.

Eating Well When You Just Can't Eat the Way You Used To. Jane Weston Wilson. New York: Workman Publishing Company, $12.95.

Everyday Health Tips. Emmaus, Pennsylvania: Rodale Press, $27.95.

Exercise as You Grow Older. Naomi Lederach, Nona Kauffman and Beth Lederach. Intercourse, Pennsylvania: Good Books, $9.95.

Heart Facts: What You Can Do to Keep a Healthy Heart. Norman K. Hollenberg, M.D., with Ilana B. Hollenberg. Glenview, Illinois: Scott Foresman, $12.95.

Maximize Your Body Potential: To An Effective Weight Management. Joyce D. Nash, Ph.D., Palo Alto. Californis: Bull Publishing Company, $14.95.

Medical and Health Guide for People Over Fifty. Eugene Nelson. Washington, D.C.: AARP Books. (See Chapter 8 for ordering AARP books.)

Prescription Drugs. by Brian S. Katcher. New York: Atheneum Publishers, $22.50.

The Surgeon General's Report on Nutrition and Health. U.S. Department of Health and Human Services and the American Nutritionists Association. New York: Warner Books, $6.95.

Financial and Retirement Planning

The Complete Retirement Planning Book. Peter A. Dickinson, $11.95 postpaid. Order from Peter Dickinson, 44 Wildwood Drive, Prescott, AZ 86301.

Finances After 50. Dorlene Shane and the United Seniors Health Cooperative. New York: Harper & Row, $10.95.

J.K. Lasser's Retirement Plan Handbook: IRAs, 401(k)s, Keoghs and Other Retirement Plans. J.K. Lasser Institute Staff. Englewood Cliffs, New Jersey: Prentice-Hall, $9.95.

Life Begins at 50, The Handbook for Creative Retirement. Leonard J. Hansen. Hauppague, New York: Barron's Educational Series, $11.95.

Medicare Made Easy. Charles B. Inlander and Charles K. MacKay, Reading, Massachusetts: Addison-Wesley, $10.95.

Money Guide to a Secure Retirement. The Editors of *Money* Magazine. New York: Oxmoor House, $13.95.

Planning Your Estate. Denis Clifford. Berkeley, California: Nolo Press, $17.95.

Retirement Edens Outside the Sunbelt. Peter A. Dickinson. Washington, D.C.: AARP Books. Order from AARP.

Retirement Places Rated. Richard Boyer and David Savageau. Englewood Cliffs, New Jersey: Prentice-Hall, $14.95.

TRAVEL

The Discount Guide for Travelers over 55. Caroline and Walter Weintz. New York: E.P. Dutton, $7.95.

Get Up And Go: A Guide for the Mature Traveler. San Francisco, California: Gateway Books, $10.95.

The Senior Citizen's Guide to Budget Travel in the U.S. and Canada. Paige Palmer. Babylon, New York: Pilot Books, $3.95.

Travel and Retirement Edens Abroad. Peter A. Dickson, 44 Wildwood Drive, Prescott, AZ, $18.50.

Travel Easy: The Practical Guide for People Over 50. Rosalind Massow. An AARP Book. Glenview, Illinoes: Scott, Foresman & Company, $8.95.

Resource Directories (Check the reference section of your local library for these volumes and others.)

Complete Guide to Prescription and Non-Prescription Drugs. H. Winter Griffith M.D., editor. Los Angeles, California: The Body Press, $19.95.

Guide to Symptoms, Illness and Surgery. Mark Pederson. Los Angeles, California: The Body Press, $14.95.

Directory of State and Area Agencies on Aging. Washington, D.C.: National Association of Area Agencies on Aging.

Encyclopedia of Senior Citizens Information Sources. Paul Wasserman, Barbara Koehler, and Yvonne Lev. Detroit: Gayle Research Company, $155.

Medical and Health Encyclopedia. Dr. Richard J. Waynman, M.D., editor. Chicago: J.G. Ferguson Publishing Co.

National Directory of Retirement Facilities. Oryx Press, $175.00. (check library or order through bookstores.)

*Resource Directory for Older People.*Superintendent of Documents. U.S. Washington, D.C.: Government Printing Office, $10.

U.S. Directory and Sourcebook on Aging. Washington, D.C.: American Association for International Aging.

MISCELLANEOUS

You're Entitled. Patrick Mayo. Bedford, New Hampshire: Linmar Associates, $9.95. A 144-page guidebook of federal government information on topics including crime protection, housing, taxes, employee protection, medical advances, travel, and veterans' programs.

The Grandparent Book. Linda B. White. San Francisco: Gateway Books, $11.95.

The Grandparenting Book. George Newman.

Grandparenting: Understanding Today's Children. David Elkind, PhD.

Grandparents and Grandchildren: The Vital Connection. Arthur Kornhaber, MD.

Oh, to Be 50 Again: On Being Too Old for a Mid-Life Crisis. Eda Leshan. New York: Time Books, Random House.

Old Age Is Not for Sissies. Art Linkletter. Viking Penguin, NY; $17.95.

Time Flies. Bill Cosby. New York: Doubleday, Dolphin Books.

FREE TO ALL PURCHASERS OF "THE MORE FOR YOUR MONEY GUIDES"

New and exciting free and deeply discounted offers are always being initiated and old ones rediscovered. To keep you informed and up-to-date on all the latest and best free offers and methods that you can take advantage of, we are offering all purchasers of our *More For Your Money Guides* a free issue of our "Best Things in Life for Free" newsletter.

Don't miss out on the newest and most innovative free opportunities available to you. Just send a self-addressed, stamped envelope to:

> "Best Things in Life for Free"
> P.O. Box 6661
> Malibu, CA. 90265

Some of the best things in life can be free! We are dedicated to providing the most fantastic, undiscovered and overloaded ideas and methods to obtain free goods, products and services for you and your family, and to alert you to the many opportunities to live, travel and enjoy life with little or no money. And, best of all, this information is free to our readers, just for asking.

Also perhaps you've also already had success with ideas of your own that have worked for you, that I haven't included in this book. If so, I would very much like to hear from you. Not only will sharing your ideas and successes be beneficial to others, but we will also pay $100 to the first person sending in an idea or method that we use in subsequent editions of our books, and $50 if it is used in our newsletter.

Additional *More For Your Money Guides* Available From Probus Publishing

Free Food ... and More, Linda Bowman,
    Order #220, $9.95

How to Go to College for Free, Linda Bowman,
    Order #219, $9.95

How to Fly for Free, Linda Bowman,
    Order #217, $9.95

Forthcoming Titles

Free Stuff for Your Pet, Linda Bowman,
    Order #271, $9.95

Free Stuff for Kids and Parents Too!, Linda Bowman,
    Order #272, $9.95

USE ORDER FORM ON NEXT PAGE TO ORDER!

ORDER FORM

Quantity	Order #	Title	Price

Payment: MasterCard/Visa/American Express accepted. When ordering by credit card your account will not be billed until the book is shipped. You may also reserve your order by phone or by mailing this order form. When ordering by check or money order, you will be invoiced upon publication. Upon receipt of your payment, the book will be shipped. Please add $3.50 for postage and handling for the first book and $1.00 for each additional copy.

Subtotal	
IL residents add 7% tax	
Shipping and Handling	
Total	

Credit Card # _____

Expiration Date _____

Name _____

Address _____

City, State, Zip _____

Telephone _____

Signature _____

Mail Orders to:

PROBUS PUBLISHING COMPANY
1925 N. Clybourn Avenue
Chicago, IL 60614

or Call:

1-800 PROBUS-1